AUTOGENIC TRAINING

AUTOGENIC TRAINING

The Effective Holistic Way
to Better Health

Dr Kai Kermani

SOUVENIR PRESS

TO EDWARD

whose vitality, enthusiasm and courage in the face of life-threatening disease inspired me to write this book, so that others in his position may use these techniques to enrich their own lives and fulfil their true potential.

Live not for the moment,
Live *the moment* with love and laughter.
                    Vernon D. Saunders

Notice to Readers

All persistent symptoms, of whatever nature, may have underlying causes that need, and should not be treated without, professional elucidation and evaluation. It is therefore very important, if you intend to use this book for self-help, only to do so in conjunction with duly prescribed conventional or other therapy. In any event, read each Part carefully, and pay particular attention to the precautions and warnings.

The Publisher makes no representation, express or implied, with regard to the accuracy of the information contained in this book, and legal responsibility or liability cannot be accepted by the Author or the Publisher for any errors or omissions that may be made or for any loss, damage, injury or problems suffered or in any way arising from the use of any methods described.

Acknowledgements

My sincere thanks to the late Drs J. W. Schultz and W. Luthe, without whom autogenic training would not have existed, for having developed and perfected the technique; to Vera Diamond, whose enthusiasm fired mine; to the late Cyril Richard and to Margaret Clark, my psychotherapists; to Judy Fraser who, although allowing my mind to wander up into the clouds, kept my feet firmly on the ground, where the technique is most needed; to Matthew Parker, for his valued contribution to the table in §2, to lesson 11 and to Appendix 1; to Ludi How for her contribution to chapter 21 on cancer; to Veda Kermani for the photographs; to Farin Dehmoubed and Farangis Kaikhosro Shahrokh for providing me with the information on Zarathustra's philosophy of life; to my optician, Terence Atkinson of Loughton, for his patience, sense of humour and unflagging attempts to improve my vision – especially when it was at its worst; to my eye specialist, Reg Daniel, for his expertise and support; to Lilla Pennent and Alayne Guarino for arranging my New York trip; and to all my patients and teachers from whom I have learnt so much. Most of all I would like to thank Edward Welch for his care, loving support and contribution to §4 on the 'rat factor'; for his invaluable help with the proof reading, and for his help with the visual aspects of this book, not least his willingness to be the subject of the photographs.

Contents

Appendices

List of illustrations and table

Preface

Many techniques and methods have been used to try to combat the unwanted effects of stress. These include Eastern forms of meditation such as transcendental and Zen, various forms of yoga, and biofeedback. The method of relaxation known as autogenic training has only relatively recently been introduced into the United Kingdom, although it was developed by Dr J. W. Schultz, a German neuropsychologist, as early as 1932, and later perfected and expanded by Dr W. Luthe in Canada. The technique used in Britain was introduced here by Dr M. Carruthers about ten years ago, and this is the version that I am going to describe in this book. AT is a simple yet powerful and effective way of relaxing, of fighting disease and disability, and of improving the quality of one's life. It has many advantages over most other techniques.

The book is written in three parts, which, for the best results, must be used in conjunction with each other.

Part 1 shows how autogenic training can be used to enhance the positive and control the negative effects of stress, and how it can enable you to utilise the immense powers inherent in stress to your best advantage, rather than allowing it to be used against you, as so often happens. It goes on to explain what AT can achieve – mentally, physically and emotionally – and the importance of being totally committed to the technique if you want to reap the full benefits. It also explains why, in the early stages, so many people encounter resistance against doing AT. Part 1 continues with a discussion of what is meant by looking after ourselves holistically, and focuses on the most important physical aspects, including good diet and nutritional supplements, which play an essential role in the perfect functioning of our total being.

Part 2 deals with the criteria that need to be satisfied and the

precautions that must be observed before undertaking autogenic training, and this is followed by step-by-step instructions on how to learn the technique **only if you do not have
access to a qualified AT trainer**. This book can also be used as
a training manual in conjunction with your trainer's instructions, provided that he or she is agreeable.

It has always been customary to learn autogenic training
from a qualified trainer. There are two main reasons why I
decided to depart from this tradition and include this section.

I have noticed, especially recently, that many inaccurate
accounts of the technique were being published in books and
magazines by people who were not properly trained and had
no intimate knowledge of its tremendous powers and the
problems that could arise if it were misused. I therefore
decided to put the record straight by writing this accurate
account. The second reason was that, following considerable
publicity for my work in catastrophic illness, especially AIDS,
I began to receive enquiries about the technique from places
as far apart as South and North America, Africa, Australia,
and even from the old Communist countries. It became
obvious to me that the only way that everyone, including
those with no access to trainers, could benefit from the
immense value and potential healing powers of AT, was to try
and reach them through this book.

Part 3 of the book covers a great many common conditions
and situations in which autogenic training has been found to
be effective – from arthritis, asthma, colitis, skin diseases and
obesity, to its uses in sport, in education and in the workplace.
For easy reference, the very diverse subjects covered here are
all listed together alphabetically. It certainly is *not* an exhaustive list – some topics have had to be left out because of lack of
space. This Part explains how various therapies (both conventional and complementary) can be combined to improve or
alleviate the various conditions discussed, and how the use of
the tremendous powers of the mind through autogenic training can maximise the effectiveness of these techniques. It
offers advice about the simple, everyday things that we can all
do to try and prevent the onset of disease, and discusses the
ways in which we can try to improve or even recover from a
troublesome condition once it has become established.

Appendix 1 covers other major therapies, both conventional and complementary, that can be used to treat or manage the various conditions dealt with. Appendix 2 gives a list of useful self-help organisations.

Autogenic training can only be maximally effective if you learn the technique stage by stage, meticulously following the instructions in Part 2, and if you practise it daily.

Finally, it is only to avoid the cumbersomeness of 'he or she', 'his or hers' and 'him or her' that I often use just 'he', 'his' and 'him'. No sexual bias is intended.

PART 1

General information for better health

§1 What is stress?

Stress is often thought of as an inevitably destructive force which can eventually lead to our physical or mental destruction. The fact is, though, that the main chemicals that are produced in the body whenever we are under stress, adrenalin and noradrenalin, are also produced in situations associated with excitement and pleasure, such as sport, competitions and sexual activity. So, clearly, life without any sort of stress would be extraordinarily boring. It is only when the stress level rises above a certain threshold, which varies from one individual to the next, that it becomes problematic and starts affecting our physical and mental well-being. This is when the symptoms associated with anxiety, depression and disturbed sleep become apparent, and we start to seek help.

In our attempt to control the symptoms, we find that tranquillisers can have an immediate and dramatic effect. But in removing the symptoms they do nothing to eradicate or control the underlying cause of the stress. The fact that thousands of tons of tranquillisers are consumed yearly all over the world, bringing about their own problems such as habituation, addiction, withdrawal reactions such as rage, and even the long-term worsening of the acute anxiety symptoms, is an indication that the use of tranquillisers, on their own, is not the answer. A great many people, including members of the medical profession, have become very alarmed at the astronomical increase in the consumption of tranquillisers, and have started to look at alternative methods of controlling stress, and, better still, of utilising it to the best advantage of the individual. For there is no doubt that excess stress plays a considerable role, directly and indirectly, in causing illness, chronic disability, morbidity and even, on occasion, death. These may range from smoking, alcoholism, depression, coronary thrombosis, strokes, nervous exhaustion and the suicide urge, to migraine, asthma, irritable bowel syndrome, colitis, stomach ulcer, chronic insomnia, cancer and even AIDS.

Furthermore, stress plays a very important role in exacerbating any serious illness that is already present. For instance, in people suffering from multiple sclerosis, cancer or AIDS the progression and spread is a great deal faster in those who are unable to control their stress level than in those who can.

Though it has been known for a long time that stress can detrimentally affect our health, it was only in the early 1970s that scientifically proven accounts of the correlation between both acute and chronic stress and disturbance of the immune system were first reported. Some of the earliest reports came from the National Aeronautics and Space Administration in the USA, where it was found that the immune systems of even such super-fit individuals as astronauts were impaired by the stress of space travel. These findings were later confirmed by numerous experiments on healthy medical students, military cadets, accountants and so on. It was found that when any such group was subjected to either chronic or acute stress, their total immunity was impaired, and it took some time for the immune system to return to normal after the stress was eliminated.

The correlation between the altered immune state, the onset of malignant disease such as cancer, and acute stress resulting from bereavement, loss of work or other threatening situation has also been well documented. It has been found that an individual under stress is much more likely to go down with cancer if he or she is of the type who is unable to deal adequately with feelings of anger, depression and frustration, and can only repress or deny them.

Early childhood deprivation may also play a part in the onset and progression of illness, as may loneliness, lack of social support, and feelings of hopelessness and helplessness. Not only is serious disease commoner in those who show a combination of these factors, but the prognosis as far as the spread of the disease is concerned is much poorer in those who accept their diagnosis resignedly and without expressing any feelings or emotions than in those who, once the initial stages of shock and denial have been worked through, put up a fight, believing that they can defeat it.

The *autonomic nervous system* controls the so-called automatic functions of the body, such as breathing, heartbeat, bowel movements, circulation, and chemical and hormonal systems, which until recently were believed to be outside our control. The sympathetic and parasympathetic are the nervous system's two main branches, and work more or less in opposite directions. The sympathetic system is responsible for the 'fight-flight' mechanism, which causes an increase in respiration, heartbeat, blood pressure and even blood cholesterol. It prepares the individual either to fight or to run away from a dangerous situation. It is basically responsible for the state of increased arousal – that dynamic state associated with stress, activity, movement and achievement.

The parasympathetic system is concerned with psycho-physiological relaxation, with recuperation after illness, and with the proper functioning of the body's internal organs. For perfect health, the two systems should be well balanced and work in harmony. THE SECRET OF MAKING STRESS WORK FOR YOU RATHER THAN AGAINST YOU IS SIMPLY TO BE ABLE TO SWITCH **at will** FROM A SYMPATHETIC-DOMINATED STATE TO A PARA-SYMPATHETIC-DOMINATED ONE, AND VICE VERSA. Autogenic training helps you to achieve this and prevents you from getting stuck in the overactive state that will eventually lead to anxiety, depression, insomnia, exhaustion or other stress-related conditions.

WHAT ARE THE THINGS IN OUR LIVES THAT WE FIND STRESSFUL?

Each one of us has to find this out for ourselves, as what may be stressful for one person may be exciting and exhilarating for another. In other words, our subjective perception colours our experience of stress. It is important not only to recognise what I shall call our own 'stressors', but also to learn to insulate ourselves against them, and this we can do via the use of autogenic training.

I mention below some of the factors that a great many people find stressful. But these are just a few guidelines, and you may or may not find your own stress-triggers here. It is important to remember that it is usually not just one stressor that causes any particular problem. Commonly, it is a com-

bination of stress-triggers, many of which may be subliminal –
that is, we may not be aware of them on a conscious level –
that can lead to trouble.

Environmental stress

This can be due either to immediate or to remote factors. The
immediate ones are numerous: a noisy workplace, problems
with one's partners or colleagues, unpleasant neighbours,
noise and air pollution due to traffic, the threat of a large
housing development next to our green-belt home, and so on.
With the advent of on-the-spot news reporting, especially on
television, we are constantly bombarded with remote environmental stressors such as famine, floods and other major
disasters. Constant reminders of the possibility of the destruction of the planet's resources through exploitation, greed and
lack of thought, and of the whole human race through nuclear
war, can also be extremely stressful. Many of us are unaware
of how these subliminal worries play on our minds, providing
a constant background of stress.

Social stress

This is triggered by interaction between the individual and
those around him: for example, wanting to date someone or to
ask someone a favour; having to fit in with other people's plans,
such as being dragged off to a party when all one wants to do is sit
quietly at home – and yet for the extrovert, having to stay at
home rather than go out and meet people can be just as stressful!
 The changing patterns of community and family life have
resulted in a lack of community and family spirit and of the
support that people used to derive from it. This, and the
ensuing loneliness can be significant sources of social stress.
Another is the isolation and stigmatisation that are forced
upon certain minority sections of society by some of those in
the majority. Take, as examples, what the Jews suffered in
Nazi Germany, and what a great many of those who are
HIV-positive or actually have AIDS are suffering now, both
openly and in more subtle ways.
 Other stressors that can be said to fall into this category are

overindulgence in alcohol; abuse of drugs, whether prescribed or obtained otherwise; overuse of chemicals such as
caffeine in coffee; or fear of the many chemicals that are now
freely used in food production.

Personal stress

This may involve the strain of relationships with immediate
members of the family, and includes such critical points in our
lives as marital breakdown, separation, divorce and even a
grown-up child leaving home. It may also involve physical
stresses, such as overstretching oneself by doing strenuous
exercise when one is not used to it; or giving birth, which, of
course, involves a great deal of emotional stresses for all
members of the family, not just the mother.

The stresses associated with any change in one's situation
or lifestyle can be quite profound. These include such things
as moving house, constant travelling, changing one's job or
partner, or even making the decision to settle down with one
particular partner. The other side of the coin – not making
enough changes in our lives, and starting to become bored,
stifled or resentful because of it – can, of course, be equally
stressful.

Another source of personal stress is the presence of acute
or chronic pain (physical, emotional or psychological), disease or disability, and the way in which other members of the
family or friends cope with this. For the person who is
seriously ill often has to deal not only with his own pain and
distress, but also with that of those around him who are
supposed to be looking after and supporting him. This is
especially difficult when he has not yet come to terms with his
own pain and distress about the situation. Emotional problems, especially if unresolved or repressed, and phobias –
such as fear of water, spiders, open or confined spaces – can
cause a great deal of stress, both overt and latent. The sexual
side of a relationship, from the point of view of demands
made as well as of frustrations and failure to satisfy each
other, especially if there is no free communication or understanding between the partners, can also be a constant source
of stress.

Work-related stress

The stresses associated with work are many and complex, ranging from those to do with commuting, boredom, lack of appreciation and overwork, to those that result from the day-to-day management of any given job, particularly decision-making. Some jobs are inherently more stressful than others – not least that of the full-time housewife, who works unlimited hours and has to deal with all the traumas of running a home, perhaps with inadequate finances, looking after not only children but perhaps a moody and demanding husband as well! For working mothers, such stresses are even harder to cope with.

These are just a few examples. You may well have different stress-triggers, and now is a good time to work out what they are, if you haven't already done so. Sit down and try and make a list of your own personal stress-triggers. This list could be invaluable in making you aware of the areas with which you have to deal in order to reduce your basic stress level.

§2　What is autogenic training?

Autogenic training, probably one of the most powerful techniques for dealing with stress that has been developed in the West, consists of a series of simple mental exercises designed to turn off the stressful 'fight-flight' mechanism in the body and turn on the restorative rhythms associated with profound psychophysical relaxation. It is a method which, when practised daily, brings about on the mental level results comparable with those achieved by Eastern meditation; and on the physical level it produces the chemical and physiological changes associated with rigorous athletic training. Unlike most other relaxation techniques, it can be practised anywhere and at any time – while travelling by train or plane, for example, in the doctor's or dentist's waiting-room, or at a disco! The time and place for practising the exercises are limited only by the imagination and the motivation of the practitioner. Some of the exercises can be practised while you are driving or walking, or in order to keep your stress level at a manageable level when you are at a meeting; or even when you are being bored by someone!

Autogenic training is particularly appealing to the Western mind, because, unlike many forms of meditation and yoga, it has no cultural, religious or cosmological overtones, and requires no special clothing or unusual postures or practices. But perhaps most important of all, as the name implies, the physical and mental relaxation, and the feelings of peace and tranquillity, are generated from within oneself and are not dependent on any external values, philosophies or therapists. Furthermore, autogenic training helps to maintain a balance between the activities of the two hemispheres of the brain, as well as between the two branches – the sympathetic and the parasympathetic – of the autonomic nervous system (page 5). AT also helps to maintain a balance between the dominant and the non-dominant halves of the brain, allowing the non-dominant half to come into its own and permit a much freer expression. The individual who is learning the technique will thus be able to get in touch with, and express freely, any latent artistic or creative flare that he may have within himself.

In a right-handed person the left (dominant) side of the brain is responsible for analytical thought, calculating, mathematical and language skills, convergent thinking and the linear mode of information processing. The right (non-dominant) side, on the other hand, is responsible for processing information and material from all sorts of different areas, including the sensory organs, which lead to intuitive interpretation and/or guesswork. It is also responsible for imaginative work, music, arts and crafts. This is the side that leads to the development of a loving, compassionate and humanitarian nature. In a left-handed person the functions of the two sides seem to vary from one individual to another.

As mentioned earlier, repression of the so-called negative emotions such as rage, anger and sadness can also cause a lot of problems as far as the inception or the progression of serious disease is concerned. Autogenic training helps us to get in touch with our true emotions and feelings and to discharge them safely and satisfactorily through specific controlled exercises, rather than repressing them and storing up trouble for future years. In the process of self-regulation, adjustment and healing that occurs during and after the practice of autogenic training, the body and the mind seem to get rid of not only present but also past stresses, memories and emotions that have not yet been fully worked through. These usually present as what are called *autogenic discharges*, in the form, for example, of temporary twitches in the muscles or of an awareness of feelings hitherto unrecognised. They usually come and go very quickly, and are completely harmless: indeed, they are an important part of the process of throwing off life's accumulated stresses. This is one of the main advantages of autogenic training: it does not cover up the cracks. On the contrary, it helps you to become aware of them and to deal with them, and thus to ensure that the peace, serenity and relaxation that you achieve are real and will remain with you. These points will be covered in greater detail in Part 2.

It is important to bear in mind that we work in stages through different levels of feelings, emotions, memories and so on. It is like peeling the layers off an onion. We work through certain things, and feel totally at peace for a while. But as we go on doing AT and working on ourselves, helping ourselves to grow, we get in touch with deeper levels, and we go through another turbulent patch. We work through that, and get on to a deeper peaceful level. Then yet more disturbance; and so on. No matter how long you have been practising AT, or any other self-growth programme, you will go through these phases. This is an integral part of true growth and of achieving a certain degree of maturity. It does not mean that AT is unsuitable for you, but that, on the contrary, it is really working, and as a result you will grow and improve, and feel much better about yourself and your life. The main reason why we seem to proceed in this stepwise fashion is that our minds have tremendous powers of self-protection and preservation, only letting us experience things, especially unpleasant ones, in small doses, so that the offloading and de-stressing process is not too uncomfortable or unpleasant for us.

ALWAYS REMEMBER THAT YOUR MIND WILL ONLY LET YOU GO AS FAR AS IT WANTS TO AND AS FAR AS IT FEELS COMFORTABLE.

Because it is such a powerful technique, **autogenic training is not suitable for everyone. So before embarking on learning it, study §8, on precautions, carefully, and make sure that you do not fall into the category of those for whom the exercises are unsuitable.**

If at all possible, learn autogenic training from a qualified trainer. This book should only be used on its own if there are no trainers close at hand. The precautions and the advice given throughout must be closely followed.

Autogenic training is usually taught individually or, preferably, in groups of six to eight, over an eight-week period. These groups are *not* psychotherapeutic and therefore no personal details or problems are discussed, though anything specific that is worrying a trainee can be discussed privately with the trainer. Each session lasts roughly two hours. The trainees are taught the positions used for the exercises, and the simple mental exercises that permit them to perform in a state of *passive concentration* as opposed to active, aim-oriented concentration. This means that the individual learns to sit back in a passive, though not resigned, way and to just observe and become aware of what happens to his mind and body after he has carried out the simple exercise commands. It is only by first becoming aware of any distress or disease in the body or mind that the mind can focus its enormous healing powers on to the distressed or diseased area and try to heal it, or to solve the problem, in the best possible way.

However, it is extremely important to realise that autogenic training is not a substitute for conventional diagnosis and therapies; it acts in conjunction with them and with complementary therapies in order to give the individual the best chance of fighting his disease or disability. If you have some physical problem, such as a bowel obstruction, that must be dealt with by conventional means. If you have acute appendicitis, no amount of AT will help that. You will still have to have surgery. But what AT does is help you to recover from the surgery a lot more quickly and satisfactorily (page 253).

The conventional or orthodox therapies are those normally used by most doctors and basically consist of chemotherapy (medications), radiotherapy and surgery. Complementary therapies (sometimes called 'alternative', a term which I personally dislike) refer to all other forms of therapies which can be used either in their own right or in combination with the conventional therapies.

Passive concentration is the simplest yet the most important concept in autogenic training. But for some individuals who are particularly used to active concentration it can be the most difficult part, though everyone manages to get into the passive state eventually (page 53).

The commands used in autogenic training are based on normal physiological sensations such as heaviness and warmth, starting from the limbs and gradually working through to one's breathing, circulation, and so on, to deep within oneself. So there is no magic or miracle about it. All that we are trying to do is to use the body's normal mechanisms and sensations in order to bypass the conscious and to get into the unconscious and the so-called silent parts of the brain, and utilise their enormous powers and energies.

PRACTICE MAKES PERFECT, AND THE MORE YOU USE AT, THE MORE YOU WILL GET OUT OF IT. **You cannot expect to get the maximum benefit from the technique if you do not commit yourself totally and use it fully and regularly.**

It is also worth remembering that you cannot expect to change overnight the bad habits and patterns of a lifetime, and certainly **AT does not work like that.** Its benefits are often imperceptible initially, and appear slowly, over a long period. If you are after a 'quick fix' or a 'magic bullet', then autogenic training is not for you and you may as well give up here and now. If, on the other hand, you want to achieve profound and long-term benefits and improvement, read on.

However powerful it may be, autogenic training is not an answer to everything. It can, though, be conveniently and harmoniously combined with a great many other therapeutic techniques, both as a starting point to get you in the right frame of mind to receive the treatment, and, later, to help enhance their effects and potential.

Table 1 shows how autogenic training can be combined with other therapies, and indicates the benefits that can ensue. A brief description of each technique and its possible applications, plus some useful addresses, are given in Appendix 1. AT combines usefully with other techniques and treatments in the following ways:

1   AT promotes a state of readiness in body and mind to benefit from whatever treatment has been chosen. It smoothes the way for that treatment to be effective.
2   The beneficial effects of treatment in the AT state are enhanced by the AT exercises.
3   In getting rid of vague aches and pains and dispersing any general feeling of unwellness, AT permits the symptoms that remain to be more easily observed and identified, with the result that diagnosis can be clearer and treatment more specific and better focused.

Table 1   How AT combines with other therapies

	These numbers refer to the numbered explanations on pp. 13 and 15.							
	1	2	3	4	5	6	7	8
Acupuncture	*	*	*	*				*
Alexander technique	*	*	*	*				*
Aromatherapy		*						*
Art therapy	*	*			*	*	*	*
Breathing therapy (rebirthing)	*	*		*			*	
Chiropractic	*	*	*				*	*
Conventional therapy	*	*	*	*			*	*
Counselling	*	*					*	*
Dance therapy (circle dancing)						*	*	
Dietary therapy		*	*					*
Flower therapy (bach remedies)	*	*	*					*
Healing	*	*						*
Herbalism	*	*						*
Homoeopathy	*	*	*				*	*
Hypnotherapy			*					*
Massage	*	*	*					*
Meditation	*	*			*		*	
Naturopathy	*	*						*

	These numbers refer to the numbered explanations on pp. 13 and 15.							
	1	2	3	4	5	6	7	8
Osteopathy	*	*	*				*	*
Polarity therapy	*	*		*				*
Reflexology	*	*						*
Shiatsu	*	*						*
Spiritual healing	*	*		*		*	*	
T'ai Chi	*	*			*	*		
Yoga	*	*		*	*	*		

4   AT integrates awareness of body and mind – physical sensations with emotional experiences and insight. So it has a good balancing effect where the chosen complementary or orthodox treatment may emphasise only one aspect of the condition.

5   AT disposes people to become open to therapies about which, irrespective of their potential value, they might have been uneasy.

6   Because AT has a balancing effect on mind and feelings and clarifies personal needs, the exercises help people to risk feeling self-conscious when starting new treatments and therapies.

7   AT exercises provide a lot of support during treatment, especially when there is an increasing awareness of feelings and of serious issues; when there is temporary muscle soreness; or when the symptoms worsen temporarily.

8   Regular performance of the AT exercises during treatment may considerably reduce the length of the treatment course.

If you are already using some other relaxation technique, keep it separate from your AT. See lesson 11 if you are already meditating.

§3 What is self-empowerment?

Self-empowerment is almost impossible to define, since its meaning varies according to each individual's perception; but although it is difficult to comprehend, it is an essential element for growth, development and transformation. I shall therefore try to explain it by describing what it means to me and by sharing some of my personal feelings and experiences with you. To me, it is the power to admit to myself my own positive attributes, as well as my inadequacies, inefficiencies and my dark side. In this way, I can acknowledge and let go of my negative and enhance my positive side. Only by doing this can I move on, transform and thus become aware of my own amazing powers to alter the course of anything, including disease and disability. This means not only reversing the detrimental physical changes that have already occurred in my body, but also preventing certain viruses such as 'flu' and other infections from getting a hold, as I have discovered over the last few years.

Some ten years ago, I was diagnosed as having a rapidly progressive condition that would eventually make me totally blind, as there was no conventional treatment for it. This prognosis proved accurate. By 1984, in spite of surgery, the vision in my right eye was completely lost. Two years later I had almost totally lost the sight in my left eye as well, and had become dependent on others. Although surgical intervention had been of no help to my right eye, I nevertheless agreed to an operation on my left eye, for this time I **knew** that surgery could be helpful. I had become aware that there was some power within me that could help me towards healing myself, and I had come to this conclusion through using not only analytical psychotherapy, but more especially autogenic training. These two therapeutic techniques also helped me to an awareness of those aspects of my life which I could not bring myself to 'look at' and 'see'. This profound awareness and the change in my mental attitude were the main differences between my first and second operations.

Since my second operation, the visual acuity in my left eye has returned to virtual normality, and that in the right eye is also returning. The night vision and the visual fields still need working on, but I am convinced that they, too, will normalise, for I am now aware of my own immense internal healing powers which I was able to tap through autogenic training, enhanced by the use of visualisations and positive affirmations while in an autogenic state of relaxation. As I became progressively more aware of my own abilities, I started using a variety of other complementary therapies, including fun, creativity, massage, reflexology and spiritual healing, and I still regularly use some of these in addition to my daily sessions of autogenic training. During the difficult time of readjustment and revaluation of my life, the unconditional love and support of those who genuinely cared for me was invaluable.

I proved the immense value of the self-healing powers gained through autogenic training for a second time when, in May 1991, I was totally blinded in the good eye following a severe penetrating injury to the eyeball. The consultant gave a hopeless prognosis because of the nature of the damage. However, using autogenics, positive affirmations and healing visualisations, I managed not only to regain my vision, but to read and write, despite having lost the mechanism for it in the accident.

It is worth bearing in mind that this combination of therapies worked for me at a particular stage of my life. Every individual and every situation that we encounter is unique, however, so it does not mean that the same combination will work for someone else, or even for me at a different point in my life. We all have to look constantly for alternatives: if one set of therapies stops working or does not work at all, it does not necessarily mean that there is anything wrong with the therapies themselves, but merely that they are not the correct ones for our current needs and circumstances.

The single most important factor for me now is the knowledge that, even if the physical improvement in my vision had not occurred, I would still have been able to live with the prospect of total blindness. The only way that I have been able to reach this state of acceptance has been by dealing with the extremely painful emotions associated with it, and this has required considerable determination and hard work. Once I had succeeded in letting go of my emotions, I could accept the idea of blindness as a lesson for my future growth and development, rather than as a misfortune sent either to punish me or to deprive me of my pleasure in life. I am convinced that, for me personally, this moment of realisation, and the transformation and wisdom that resulted, signalled the start of the process of healing in its true holistic sense. I now know that there will never come a time when I shall be able to slacken off and feel that the work on myself has been completed. We must realise that once we embark on such a journey, it is a never-ending one.

Remember that there is nothing special or unique about me. I have seen the same sort of changes, healing and remission occur in other individuals suffering from serious or catastrophic diseases (see list of conditions in Part 3 – even potentially fatal ones like cancer (p. 185) and AIDS (p. 158) – provided that the affected individuals were aware of their own capabilities and could put their shoulders to the grindstone and work hard to overcome their illness.

If we manage to start on this journey of change and transformation, we inevitably become aware of the existence of unconditional love for ourselves and others. There is nothing wrong with loving ourselves in the purest sense of the word; an empty, drained-out battery cannot give out any energy. In the same way, we cannot give love if we do not love ourselves. It is by loving ourselves and thus enriching our own lives that we can act as a light and energy source for others who may come into contact with us, and the more love we give the more we shall receive. I strongly believe that the awareness of the presence of this love deep within us is an absolute prerequisite for healing in the true holistic sense to occur.

Achieving this goal is very difficult and requires constant hard work – even more when we are trying to apply the same principles to people for whom we care greatly. This state of unconditional love, and the peace and tranquillity which may be associated with it, seem to come in stages, and I don't think that we ever reach a point in our lives when we can honestly say that we feel unconditional love in every situation and for everyone we meet. For that to happen, we would have to reach a state of perfection which is impossible for most of us as mortal human beings, with all our imperfections and our dark side. However, we can at least strive to get as near to that state as possible by acknowledging every misfortune that befalls us and letting go of all the distress associated with it. The problems we encounter may be related to our sexuality, religious upbringing, social conditioning and taboos; fears of various sorts including pain, whether it be physical, emotional, psychological or spiritual; fear of disease, disability, loss and, in its ultimate form, dying and death. Not only must we be aware of them, acknowledge and own them, but we must try to work with them, so that we can open out and clarify our own lines of communication and our own channels. Unless we do that, we shall never become aware of our own strength and power.

We can all help the sick individual to empower himself, irrespective of whether we are professional carers, friends or relatives. We can do this by being passive, accepting and non-judgemental, realising that his empowerment has nothing to do with us. All that we hope to do is to provide a safe haven for him to do his own work and, if he feels so inclined, to draw upon his own immense internal powers and move on. This can take a long time and may require a great deal of patience and loving support, since each individual will go at his own pace – the pace that is comfortable for him but which may be totally wrong and uncomfortable for us. But we must not push our own speed or project our own needs on to him – this is extremely important. We should just be there and allow the individual to exercise his own options. The choice is always his, and we can only act as a guide to show him the various paths that may be available to him. We must be very careful not to project our own negative and unresolved conflicts onto him, but remain steadfast and clear, mirroring all the superb qualities that lie dormant within him; all the love, care, compassion, strength, dignity and power. We all have such qualities within us, but unfortunately most of the time their clarity is dimmed by the superficial feelings of self-doubt, guilt, shame, worthlessness and inadequacy which are too readily exploited by others wishing to see only our negative side.

Apart from using specific therapeutic tools and techniques,

we as carers can help sick individuals to recover from disease and fight disability by giving them loving support, hope, confidence, and the knowledge that there is indeed an enormous reservoir of untapped resources within themselves that they can fall back on at times of difficulty and hardship. For without such hope, without a goal or a purpose, without a belief and faith in our own strength, power and capabilities, there is little left to fight for – and fight we all must, constantly, against a whole range of events which will wage a war of attrition against us if allowed to get out of hand. We must not become despondent or lose heart, especially at times when we feel that everything is against us and nothing seems to be going right. These are the times when we are being truly tested. Dr Elisabeth Kübler-Ross, who is well known for her work in the field of dying and death, says, 'If the canyons were sheltered from the storm, we would never see the beauty of their carvings.' In her wisdom, Nature may sometimes bend us to what seems an intolerable extent, but she will never break us. The bendings and contortions and what seem like very unfair events are only our lessons towards growth, maturity, transformation and healing; we must accept them as such and not think of them as vengeful punishment for past misdeeds; nor should we feel that we deserve what has been doled out to us, because we are unworthy individuals.

We can all achieve our aims, whatever they may be, by accepting ourselves as whole, complete, unique, loving and lovable individuals – which indeed we are, disease and disability included. By doing this, and by acknowledging our negative as well as our positive attributes, we can reach beyond the confining and paralysing fear of disability, disease and death, to the dawn of awareness of our full healing potential. It is imperative to realise that no one else can do this for us, although we need others to show us the way and guide us along, especially when we hit the hard, difficult and painful patches or the blind alleys. It is up to us and our inner wisdom to do the best for ourselves. This necessarily entails a fine balance between intuition and experience, which can be achieved by the use of a technique such as autogenic training.

It is extremely important to remember that no matter how positive, enlightened or tranquil we may feel at any moment, these are only comparatively transient states, as are the negative and oppressive feelings we may get from time to time. We are bound to oscillate constantly between them, especially at the beginning of our journey of change, as we will between the new, unfamiliar and often scary patterns of behaviour and thought, and the old, familiar ones that may feel a lot safer. There is absolutely nothing wrong in that, so long as we are aware of what is going on and make a conscious decision about which state we wish to dwell in at any particular time. Hopefully, every time we step out of the old, often unproductive and destructive patterns, the onward journey towards newer and better ones will become that much easier. This is all part and parcel of the process of growth, transformation and empowerment. As most of us are not saints, we should not expect the impossible from ourselves; we should not become despondent and feel that we have failed if we decide to rest our weary beings somewhere familiar for a while. This journey of transformation and its consequent empowerment is hard work and at times exhausting. Provided that we have set our sights on change, however, the thrust of our journey will be forever forward, and with every step of the way we shall be able to reclaim that much more inherent power, strength and dignity that could be within our grasp, if only we would reach out for it.

Apart from using this power to fight disease and disability, there are other ways in which we can utilise it. Our mother earth, who for so long has nurtured and cared for us despite being mercilessly polluted and having her resources so uncaringly and unthinkingly plundered, is facing devastation and destruction. The choice for the survival of our planet is simple and stark: we either abrogate our responsibilities and allow ourselves to be overcome by gloom and despondency and washed away by the flood of despair and depression, or we rise up to the challenge. We can voice our dismay at what is going on, accept our responsibility boldly and courageously and join with others who are fighting for an improvement in our environment. In so doing, we can also meet those who are less privileged than ourselves and need our help, lightening their load and helping them out of the dark abyss of poverty, starvation, disease, disability and despair and back into the light, while celebrating, affirming and reaffirming the joyous gifts of love and life.

§4 The 'rat factor'

By 'rat' I mean the resistance that so many people encounter
in themselves against doing autogenic training in the early
stages ('rat' = resistance to AT!). In fact, RESISTANCE IS RIFE
WHENEVER WE UNDERTAKE ANYTHING THAT IS DIFFERENT, OR
INVOLVES CHANGES IN OURSELVES OR OUR OUTLOOK, OR GROWTH
IN THE BROADEST SENSE OF THE WORD.

One of the main reasons for resistance has to do with our
reticence to put ourselves first and give ourselves the time and
space just to be with ourselves. If we fail to do this in the early
stages, a kind of 'Catch 22' situation can arise, and we may
become frustrated and convince ourselves that we are wasting
our time. The resistances, and the activities of what we might
call the 'dirty tricks department', which is responsible for the
activities of the 'rat', take many forms. This section is designed to help you, the trainee, to identify the often very
subtle ways that these resistances can make themselves felt.
After you have learned to recognise them for what they are –
mere distractions – you will be in a better position to deal with
them when they arise. It is important to remember, though,
that resistances are *not* all bad. They can act as a block to
prevent you from moving too fast or too deeply within
yourself before you are ready to deal with whatever package
you may be carrying around with you that needs to be sorted
out or cleaned up!

One of the most common remarks made by trainees during
the first few weeks of training is that they find the trainer's
voice very soothing and relaxing. 'Is it possible for me to have
a tape of it?', they ask. This is a very clear indication of the 'rat
factor' at work. The trainee is quite happy to attend the
training sessions and listen to the voice of a total stranger
doing all the work and 'permitting' him to relax, but when it
comes to getting down to it himself and giving himself permission to relax, then he finds a whole plethora of reasons and

excuses for not getting on with his exercises regularly. The response to the request for a tape must be an emphatic *No!* (And you should see some of the hurt expressions.) Later on when he has grown more accustomed to the special phrases (§10) and has found his own rhythm and his own internal voice, he will start to resent the intruding voice of the therapist and will want to continue on his own. This should be encouraged right from the beginning, as it will help the trainee to empower himself to become responsible for his own care and well-being.

For those of you who have no access to any qualified therapist or trainer, and who are entirely dependent on this book for learning the technique, the problem is quite different. As you will depend exclusively on your own efforts right from the beginning, the great temptation will be to leave your exercises until later, to skip through the lessons in any old order, or, most commonly of all, to allow insufficient time between the lessons and to try to rush through the whole thing. This would be the prime example of the dirty tricks department, or the 'rat', at work, as it would inevitably prevent you from delving very deeply into the process and thus from gaining the maximum benefit.

Resistance is often particularly strong in this context, and can take a number of forms, ranging from the sublime to the truly inspired! It no longer surprises me to hear trainees say, for instance, that since they were on holiday during the last fortnight they had to miss out their exercises! And it is amazing how washing the dishes, painting the kitchen, or any other chores that we normally dislike, come suddenly within the orbit of the dirty tricks department. Catching up on a bit of letter-writing and having to make that important telephone call or cup of tea also seem to be quite popular get-outs! Everybody who has done, or ever will do, AT will experience these distractions in one way or another. And the longer they do it, the more astounded they will become at their immense range and subtlety; no matter how long we go on practising the technique, we should always be on the look-out for the 'rat factor'.

Another very common indication of the 'rat' at work is a trainee's report that halfway through the exercises he experienced visual phenomena with his eyes closed. Sometimes these appear like short filmstrips or extracts from television commercials. Auditory disturbance may also occur, so that a refrain from a familiar song or jingle can begin to repeat itself *ad infinitum*, causing confusion and frustration. This is very tiresome, and usually means that the trainee has to terminate the exercise before coming to the end. Other forms of resistance include intruding, often unimportant, thoughts, such as 'What am I going to cook for supper tonight?' or 'What train should I take?'. The range is endless, and you will come across them more frequently than you would wish! The important thing is to be aware of what is going on and to bring your attention back to the task in hand. It is a good idea, though, to think about what the possible reasons for the intrusion may have been. Whatever the cause, one thing is certain. Such distractions interfere with your relaxation and prevent you from going very deeply within yourself and thus from getting the most out of your autogenic training.

Other forms of resistance are associated with laziness and lack of motivation. This is quite a common form of resistance initially, for although we may kid ourselves that we are highly motivated and very much want to improve ourselves, deep down inside we may not be really ready for it, or else we are afraid of the transformation that may occur in us. No matter how bad our current predicament may be, at least we know the rules of the game. However, if we change, if we move on into new areas and ventures, it will be almost like starting from scratch or like entering a foreign territory whose rules are totally unknown to us. It is important to accept this situation if it arises, and to realise that we can only change at the rate that is comfortable for us. Furthermore, as we proceed on our journey of growth, improvement and empowerment, the transformation will not be easy and there are bound to be times, especially when we are going through a particularly difficult patch, when we get scared, regress or even wonder why on earth we are doing these things to improve and change ourselves. This is part and parcel of growth and maturity. The most important thing at these times of difficulty, doubt and pain is to accept all our shortcomings and keep our sights firmly fixed on our goal of growth and improvement. By so doing, we will find that, with time, patience and help, we are able to work through these problems and resistances, and let the 'rat' rest, at least for a while. He is bound, though, to become highly active from time to time, as we proceed on our journey of growth, self-discovery and self-realisation.

One other major problem which may be associated with our new growth and maturity is the fact that our transformation can be very threatening, even unacceptable, to those close to us, who may not be at the same stage of the journey or, indeed, on the same road at all. This may cause difficulties and external pressures, as well as activating the 'rat' internally. If such problems arise, it is very important that those involved discuss them freely, even if it means enlisting the help of a professional therapist. It would be a great pity if we had to forgo our transformation and self-empowerment because of domestic problems which could easily have been overcome with a modicum of thought and discussion. Twitching muscles, involuntary jerks, yawning, pain and nerve spasm, and other physical manifestations can also intrude, as well as emotional and psychological distractions such as tuning in to past feelings of sadness, happiness or anger. These forms of autogenic discharge, which often indicate a need to offload some of the repressed and unresolved emotions and memories that the trainee may be carrying (lesson 5), are fully discussed in Part 2.

This chapter has described just some of the ways in which resistances may present themselves in their effort to interefere with your progress towards improvement, self-realisation and self-empowerment. You will find out exactly how to deal with them in Part 2. **But the most important thing is to be aware of the tricks of the mind and the activities of the 'rat'**, for once you are wise to their antics, you are more than halfway towards being able to do something about them!

§5 Holistic health

Some people have very bizarre ideas about *holism*, because they think that the word comes from 'holy'. In fact it comes from 'whole', so the accent is on completeness. I see holism as a way of looking at the various aspects of the body, mind, emotions and spirit equation, and doing something about improving each of these aspects. Each is commonly known as a *quadrant*, as usually in this context the whole person is represented as a circle, and each of the four aspects as a quarter (quadrant) of the circle.

Currently in the West, unfortunately, we are not encouraged to lead a balanced life by working on all four quadrants and developing them equally. Most of us have developed at least one quadrant at the expense of the others. For instance, take someone like me. Highly educated, I had depended on the marked overdevelopment of my intellectual capacities without due regard to any of the other aspects for a considerable part of my life – certainly for all the time that I was studying. It is only during the last few years that I have become aware of my deficiencies in the other quadrants, and have made a strenuous effort to redress the balance by working on those other quadrants in the hope of improving the quality of my life and making it much richer, fuller and worthwhile in all aspects, rather than in just one or two.

I BELIEVE THAT IN THE TRUE HOLISTIC APPROACH TO HEALTH AND TO THE MANAGEMENT OF DISEASE THERE MUST BE A HAPPY AND HARMONIOUS RELATIONSHIP BETWEEN THE ORTHODOX METHODS AND THE BEST OF THE COMPLEMENTARY TREATMENTS. ONE SET OF TREATMENTS SHOULD NOT BE USED AT THE EXPENSE, OR TO THE EXCLUSION, OF THE OTHER. All may have a part to play in the management of the sick person, and it should be for him or her to decide which therapy he or she wishes to use, once all the pros and cons of the particular treatments available have been pointed out honestly and openly, with the benefit of all the current knowledge. For after all, the sick person is much more likely to be aware of his inner wisdom and requirements than anyone else. And we must always be alert to the fact that 'one man's meat may be another man's poison'.

Aspects of the physical side of holistic medicine include exercise, diet, nutritional supplements, and the avoidance of tobacco, alcohol and other stimulant non-prescribed or recreational drugs. I will not go into these aspects in great detail, as there are already numerous books available, some of which are mentioned in the Further Reading list at the end of this book. However, I am going to mention a few points about each, which are paticularly important. (These aspects are fully discussed in §6.)

The importance of the *mind* and the *emotions* and the stress inherent in the latter have already been mentioned in §1. It is important, in order to deal with repressed emotions, that these two quadrants are properly and truthfully acknowledged and dealt with by means of a technique or techniques which are acceptable and appropriate to the individual, whether it be autogenic training or some other therapy involving deep relaxation. Other techniques which may be suitable in this context are individual or group therapy, of which there are a great many varieties. These include psychotherapy, transactional analysis, psychosynthesis, counselling and co-counselling (see Appendix 1). The mind and the emotions are discussed in greater detail in Part 2.

As soon as *spirituality* is mentioned, some people either freak out or switch off because of some very basic misconceptions about the subject – particularly because of the mistaken belief that 'spiritual' and 'religious' mean the same. Some people are able to combine the two, but it does not have to be so. You do not need to believe in God to believe in spirituality. Some also believe that a spiritual experience is a bizarre or cosmic experience that happens out of the blue or appears from outer space, suddenly and unexpectedly. This is not normally the case. As far as I am concerned, a spiritual experience is that deep and satisfying joy and contentment that I derive from something as simple as a beautiful flower or a glorious summer's day. Some get the same feeling from helping a friend or relation in distress, doing voluntary work, or even from their work or profession. I have had some of the most exhilarating and stimulating experiences of my life while taking individuals ill with cancer or AIDS through autogenic training courses, and watching their extraordinary courage in their fight to extend, and to improve the quality of, their lives. To be involved in their growth and transformation has been a spiritual experience for me.

It is important to bear in mind that we can and do have spiritual experiences throughout our daily lives. Most of us are unaware that these experiences are indeed spiritual, and so are unable to draw upon their tremendously uplifting and enlivening powers, especially at times of hardship, serious disease or disability. All that we have to do is become aware of these experiences and acknowledge them; for once we allow ourselves to do this, we will find ourselves getting in touch with, and thus being able to draw upon, an immense source of power and energy that usually lies dormant within us.

I find the teachings of Zarathustra (also known as Zoroaster) of great interest in this context. He was a philosopher and religious leader who lived in Iran more than 2,500 years ago. He advocated that we should respect and cherish not only our fellow human beings, but also the animal, plant and mineral kingdoms. He also maintained that whatever gifts we may be endowed with are not purely for our own personal benefit, but are to be used in the service of others in trying to help those less fortunate than ourselves at every level of body, mind, emotions and spirit. We should aim during our lifetime towards the ultimate wisdom, knowledge, altruism, purity, love and truth. For it is only by so doing that we can create a harmonious, peaceful and loving home on this planet for every kind of life that inhabits it. The basis of his teachings can be summarised in three very important and profound phrases: *good thoughts*, which necessarily lead to *good words* and *good deeds*.

§6 Exercise, diet, nutritional supplements and other physical factors

EXERCISE

I have not yet come across any specific references to the relationship between exercise and the immune system, but we know that exercise definitely changes the chemistry and physiology of the body towards better health, in addition to making us feel good, relaxed and happy. These sensations are probably associated with the release of a number of useful chemicals, including endorphins, into the blood when we exercise. Endorphins are naturally occurring morphine-like substances, which probably account for the well-being that is associated with doing sport.

It is very important, though, to **exercise within your capabilities**, especially if you have not exercised before or for a long time. But most important of all, you should **really enjoy what you decide to do**, for unless you enjoy the sport that you have picked you will not be able to continue with it for long. Don't try to push yourself beyond your limit. You don't really have to do a five-mile jog or an hour's hard work-out at the gym to benefit from exercise! Usually, gentle, rhythmic exercises are better than those that require sudden bursts of energy such as sprinting. Swimming is excellent, if you happen to like water! A brisk walk is also a fine way of getting the muscles and circulation on the move. Creative movements, dance and meditative movements can all be of great benefit. Find the one that gives you the maximum pleasure, as well as fitness (see Appendix 1). If you are unable to do any of these, just do a few minutes' gentle stretching exercises. But whatever you decide to do, be gentle with yourself and don't overdo it. Listen to your body, and if it objects by giving you pain or any other symptoms, respect that objection and modify your exercise routine accordingly.

DIET

The building blocks of the body, and our main source of
energy, are derived from the food that we eat. Since food is
thus the basic sustainer of life, it is extremely important to pay
close attention to it. Let's look at it this way. If you had a very
expensive car designed to take 5-star petrol, but instead of
5-star you continually put in 1- or 2-star, how long do you
think it would go on functioning properly? Not very long, I am
sure.

Our bodies are the most complex and delicate machines
ever created. It is therefore astonishing how little attention
we pay to the sort of fuel that we put into them. I marvel at
how long our long-suffering bodies go on functioning perfectly with hardly a complaint, despite the rubbish that we
pour in and the way we abuse them over the years. It is
important to realise that the information that I give here,
especially that concerning diet and nutritional supplements,
can only be a guideline, since detailed discussion is well
outside the scope of this book. There are numerous books on
the market devoted to all aspects of the body and how they
can be improved, and a few useful books are included in the
Further Reading list. Obviously, it pays to feed ourselves with
food of the best quality at all times. However, we must be
realistic, and recognise that, for whatever reason, the ideal
cannot always be attained. It is important that we should be
aware when our diet is inadequate, so that we can add the
necessary supplements.

There are probably as many diets as there are days in the
year! So I am not going to recommend any particular ones,
especially since different individuals will have different
needs, as well as likes and dislikes. But I will make a few basic
general points, which hopefully will make choosing your diet
a bit easier. ·

**The diet that you choose must be simple, nutritious, practical
and, above all, enjoyable.** For if it does not satisfy all these
criteria you will find it very difficult to stick to it for long. It
must include plenty of fresh fruit, vegetables, whole grains
and fibre. (For advice about many specific conditions, see
relevant sections in Part 3.) Try, whenever you can, to use

fruit and vegetables raw, or as lightly cooked (preferably steamed) as possible, so that the maximum goodness is preserved and not destroyed by overcooking. Don't forget to have plenty of protein, for it also provides, as well as a lot of energy, a great variety of basic nutrients, including supplements. If you are a traditional eater, try to stick to white meats such as chicken, turkey and fish whenever you can. The red meats may be nice to eat, but they are often very fatty; even the leanest fillet steak can contain as much as 15 per cent fat, as well as a number of chemicals and hormones that are used to increase the yield of the animal. As you probably know, animal fats are unhealthy, especially as far as the build-up of cholesterol is concerned, since that can lead to atherosclerosis (hardening of the arteries), which in turn leads to poor circulation, coronaries and strokes.

If you decide to go completely vegetarian, do study the subject carefully or consult a qualified dietitian, so that you do not become deficient in anything, especially first-class proteins, which are the essential building blocks of almost all of the body's chemicals, hormones and enzymes, as well as providing muscle and energy. Don't forget to replace the animal proteins such as meat and eggs with nuts, grains and pulses.

NUTRITIONAL SUPPLEMENTS

Supplements are substances that are essential for the proper functioning of our bodies, and may or may not be present in tiny amounts in the food that we eat daily. Some supplements are particularly important for the proper functioning of the immune system, and these can be particularly scarce in our diets. I discuss briefly here only the most important ones, under the headings of vitamins, amino acids and trace elements. (They are all fully discussed in books listed in the Further Reading section.)

Vitamins

All vitamins are necessary for the normal functioning of the body. Most people on well balanced diets get sufficient amounts of them during the day. However, if the diet is inadequate or unbalanced, then some vitamins may not be available and may lead to certain deficiencies. The story of lack of vitamin C causing scurvy in the mariners of old is a classic one. An obvious situation in which the body's vitamin requirements increase is when a person is suffering from some chronic and debilitating disease. This may be due to inadequate absorption of vitamins from the gut in certain stomach and bowel disorders, or there may be an unusually heavy demand for them at times when the body is trying to manufacture certain chemicals that it is not producing enough of. Such a situation can arise even in normal states such as pregnancy, when the requirement for all substances is considerably increased in order to cater for the growing baby as well as the mother. The need for increased amounts of iron to correct anaemia is also well known.

It is important to remember that, like every other dietary component, vitamins should be taken in the correct recommended doses; for overdoses can cause side effects, some of which can be quite serious.

For anyone who just wants to supplement his diet to ensure that he is getting sufficient amounts of vitamins, one of the multivitamin preparations with trace elements, stocked by chemists and healthfood shops, is usually enough. Remember when you are buying them that cost is not necessarily a guide to the quality of the product. Read the label to see what is inside each tablet or capsule, and compare it with competing products. Choose the one that gives you the best value for money.

Vitamin A   This vitamin is fat-soluble and so can be stored and accumulated in the body. It is therefore important *not* to exceed the stated dose as side effects can ensue. It is found in such substances as carrots, fish liver oil, liver, green and yellow vegetables, eggs, milk and dairy products, margarine and yellow fruits. In certain conditions such as AIDS and cancer the requirement for vitamin A is greatly increased, to about 10,000–25,000 international units daily, and it should preferably be taken in the form of betacarotene, which is much safer than vitamin A, in the dose of 12,500 international units once or twice a day, or up to a maximum of three times a day.

The vitamin B group   I mention the members of the B group together because they usually enhance each other's benefits, and because in most supplements they are present together in the correct amounts. Some B vitamins have specific functions – for instance, B12 for pernicious anaemia and B6 for pre-menstrual and menopausal symptoms – which I will refer to in greater detail in specific sections of Part 3. They are all water-soluble and are not stored in the body, and therefore have to be taken daily. The best natural sources are yeast, bran, whole wheat, peanuts, pork, most vegetables, fish, eggs and cheese.

Vitamin C   This is also a water-soluble vitamin which is not stored in the body so has to be taken regularly. The main sources are fresh fruit and vegetables, especially citrus fruits, tomatoes and potatoes.

Requirements vary considerably: for routine maintenance, up to 1 gram a day, depending on other natural sources consumed. Those suffering from chronic and debilitating diseases such as AIDS or cancer may require much larger doses: anything from 1 to 6 grams daily, depending on individual tolerance and side effects. Remember that in some people even small doses can cause stomach ache or diarrhoea. If that is the case, it is best to take the vitamin in small doses throughout the day, and preferably in the soluble forms, which have been specially formulated to be as near to neutral as possible.

Vitamin D   This is a fat-soluble vitamin, and the best sources are natural sunlight, fish liver oils, sardines, herrings, tuna, salmon, milk and dairy products. The normal dose is from 400 to 1000 international units a day.

Vitamin E   The best natural sources are wheatgerm, soya beans, vegetable oils, broccoli, sprouts and spinach, whole wheat and other whole grains, and eggs. The normal daily dose of vitamin E varies from 100 to 1000 international units daily, and it may be supplied in conjunction with certain trace elements such as selenium, as they work together better (see page 35).

Amino acids

These are the building blocks for the manufacture of protein in the body. Without them, most of the body's systems, including the immune system, which is vital for maintaining health, cannot function properly. Of the twenty-two known amino acids, eight are referred to as 'essential', and if they are absent, even temporarily, from the diet – and they cannot be manufactured by the body – protein deficiency and malfunctioning of organs and body systems soon ensue. The main sources of these important substances are animal and vegetable proteins, such as meat, poultry, fish and soya beans, peanuts, milk and cheese. Soya beans are one of the best sources, as they contain all the essential amino acids.

Although individual amino acids are available, for general purposes – if a supplement is required – it is best to take one of the prepared compounds, which are finely balanced. And it is advisable to take vitamin supplements at the same time, as amino acids and vitamins complement and enhance each other's functions. An amino acid supplement is not usually required by people who eat a normal, well balanced diet. But it may be required by those with chronic wasting diseases such as AIDS or cancer, or by those who have problems with digesting or absorbing amino acids. Two amino acids, arginine and lysine, are of particular importance to anyone suffering from *herpes* (see pages 216–18).

Trace elements

These are substances found only in minute amounts in a few foods. Except for a few well known ones, like iron, their extremely important function in the body's metabolic processes, including those of the immune system, was not appreciated until relatively recently.

Calcium This is essential for the proper building and maintenance of bones and teeth, and for the functioning of the cardiovascular (heart and circulation) system. The main sources are milk, cheese, green vegetables, sardines, salmon and soya beans. The daily requirement is about 800–1500 mg, but it can be considerably more during periods of growth, recovery from fractures, and during the menopause (see §36, §48).

Iron A deficiency of this element leads to anaemia, which is particularly prevalent in women during their reproductive period and pregnancy, and in the elderly. The main natural sources are liver, kidney, red meat, egg yolk, oatmeal and spinach. There is a wide variety of preparations, and the dose will vary depending on the one used. So be guided by the manufacturer's recommendations.

Magnesium This element seems to be helpful in osteoporosis (thinning of bones) and symptoms of pre-menstrual syndrome. The best naturally occurring sources are cocoa, chocolate, seafood (winkles, whelks and shrimps), nuts (cashews, brazils and almonds), grains (barley and wheat), and some vegetables, particularly beans, peas and spinach beet. The normal daily requirement is about 6 mg per kilogram of body weight, or roughly 350 mg for men and 300 mg for women.

Selenium The importance of this element has been discovered only relatively recently, and one of its main functions seems to be to enhance the functioning of the immune system. Its main natural sources are wheatgerm, bran, tuna, onions, tomatoes and broccoli. Most healthy people get their requirements largely from normal foods, but those who are seriously ill need an additional supplement of 100–300 micrograms daily. Selenium is best taken in combination with vitamins A, C and E, as they improve its absorption.

Zinc This element seems to oversee the proper functioning of a great many of the body's essential systems. It can be present in small amounts in lamb, pork, wheatgerm, yeast and eggs. As a supplement, it is usually available in the form of zinc sulphate and zinc gluconate tablets, in doses ranging from 15 to 300 mg a day. These combination salts seem to be equally effective, though zinc gluconate seems to be better tolerated. Doses for sulphate and gluconate are different, so follow the manufacturer's recommendations and do not exceed them, as too much zinc can cause side effects.

'RECREATIONAL' DRUGS

It is a well known fact that both **smoking and drinking alcohol can cause severe physical and mental problems**, particularly if practised in excess and over a long period. The amount of damage they can cause seems to vary from one person to another, so the best thing to do is to try to **avoid them altogether**; or if that is not possible, **cut down to an absolute minimum. It is of the utmost importance, if you want to remain healthy, to avoid at all costs** the other so-called recreational drugs such as marijuana (hashish), but particularly narcotics such as cocaine and its derivatives, morphine and heroin.

SAFER SEX

The final item on the physical level that is worth mentioning here is **the avoidance of unprotected (by condom, or sheath) penetrative sex with a casual partner, whether between man and woman or man and man.** For the condom can prevent you from catching not only the ordinary sexually transmitted diseases such as syphilis, gonorrhoea and NSU (non-specific urethritis), but also HIV infection which can lead to AIDS. It is worth bearing in mind that it is possible to catch gonorrhoea during oral sex with a person who has no symptoms but is nonetheless infected – a point which is often overlooked. DO REMEMBER THAT YOU CAN HAVE AS MUCH FUN BY OTHER MEANS SUCH AS TOUCH AND MASSAGE, WITHOUT HAVING PENETRATIVE SEX, WITH A CASUAL OR UNKNOWN PARTNER. YOU JUST NEED TO USE YOUR IMAGINATION AND INTUITION A BIT MORE!

PART 2

Autogenic training, step by step

§7 How do I use Part 2?

It is extremely important to read the early sections in Part 2, particularly the precautions and preliminaries, before going any further. Also reread page 11.

Decide whether you are going to spend **one or two weeks** on each exercise or set of exercises – that is, on each lesson.

Read through only one exercise at a time. Do the exercises regularly, and unless directed otherwise, only move on to the next if you have mastered the one that you have just been learning. Remember that the exercises are **cumulative** – that is, new instructions are always added to what you have learned before. Lessons 1 to 4 and 6 to 8 are added to each other week by week. There is one exception to this, however. Although the *offloading exercises* are not described until lesson 5, which is where we usually introduce them, if at any time during the earlier exercises you get in touch with un-resolved feelings, emotions or memories, do turn to page 85 and use the offloading exercises freely, as they can be of enormous value not only in helping you with your autogenic training exercises, but also in making you feel better if repressed emotions are one of your problems.

GET YOURSELF A SMALL NOTEBOOK, so that you can keep a record of the exercises and chart your progress during the next few weeks. You only need to make brief notes of the most salient points. Please **do make sure that you write immediately after each exercise**; otherwise, you will forget what you have experienced very quickly.

Make a list of both your short-term and your long-term objectives, including what you hope to achieve from doing AT, and what parts of your life, yourself and/or your personality you wish to change, modify or improve. By the time you have learnt the technique properly, you will be able to set about achieving your aims.

Be sure to use all four main AT positions, described in §9.

§8 Precautions: when not to undertake autogenic training

I mentioned earlier that although autogenic training is a simple technique, it is a very powerful one and may not, therefore, be suitable for everyone. **Learn the method from a qualified trainer**, if at all possible. **Only use this book as your teacher if there are no qualified trainers within easy reach.** If this is the case, **it is imperative that you read the following paragraphs particularly carefully. Do not undertake autogenic training in any of the following circumstances:**

1 **During or immediately following a heart attack (acute myocardial infarction).** AT is extremely helpful if it is undertaken about three months after a heart attack, as it can help to prevent possible heart problems in the future. It is also very useful in trying to combat, OR PREVENT, cardiac neurosis – the fear of carrying on with a normal life in case one might have another heart attack – that may afflict anyone who has already had one. However, if anyone who is a regular user of the technique suffers from a heart attack, they can continue using it to improve symptoms and speed up recovery.

In addition, it is quite helpful for those suffering from the kind of chest pains that are produced after exertion (Angina, page 164), as it tends to improve the general circulation of the body and so, hopefully, will improve the circulation to the heart and relieve the condition.

If, for whatever reason, you have irregular heartbeats, you should undertake AT with caution, and must certainly leave out lesson 4 (the heartbeat exercise). It would not do you any harm, but it could be uncomfortable and off-putting if you were to get in touch with an irregular heartbeat.

2 **If you are a diabetic undergoing insulin treatment**, as insulin consumption and utilisation alters considerably while doing AT and therefore needs constant blood and urine monitoring, which is not usually possible for the majority of diabetics.

3 **If you suffer from glaucoma** (increased pressure within the eyeball), though AT can be very effective in reducing the pressure, **provided** that the pressure is regularly checked to ensure that it does not rise further as it sometimes can do.

4 **If you suffer from psychotic conditions such as schizophrenia, or severe depression associated with hallucinations or feelings of unreality.**

5 **If you have had electric shock treatment** (ECT).

6 **If you are an active alcoholic or drug abuser** – using hard drugs such as heroin, morphine, cocaine, crack – as you may experience severe feelings of withdrawal as well as depression, not to mention the fact that you will not be in a fit mental state or have sufficient motivation to do the exercises every day.

However, autogenic training can be undertaken after you have 'dried out', or when you have been off hard drugs for at least six months. If this applies to you, you may find the offloading exercises (lesson 5) for the release of pent-up and repressed emotions particularly helpful. However, if despite using these exercises you still make contact with uncomfortable or unpleasant sensations or feelings, stop practising autogenic training and seek the help of a counsellor or therapist, who should be able to help you to deal with them.

IF YOU ARE ADDICTED TO TRANQUILLISERS OR SLEEPING TABLETS YOU ARE A VERY SUITABLE CANDIDATE FOR AUTOGENIC TRAINING, as it will help you to cope not only with your anxieties, and even their underlying causes, but also with the withdrawal effects. AT is probably one of the most effective hypnotics (sleep-inducers).

7 **If you suffer from epilepsy.** Although AT can be helpful for people with this condition, occasionally it can increase the frequency of attacks. It is therefore advisable that you do **not** undertake training if you suffer from epilepsy.

8 **If, for any reason, you have had a prolonged episode of unconsciousness.**

If you do not fall into any of these categories, then you are a suitable candidate for autogenic training, and you can proceed.

§9 Preliminaries: exercise positions and other essentials

There are certain essential preparations that you have to make before you can proceed any further. So it is very important that you read this chapter carefully and note the instructions and advice that are given.

Having read the previous sections, paying particular attention to §8, you now know whether you are a suitable candidate for autogenic training. Assuming that you are, and that you would like to learn the technique, you must decide first of all over how long a period you wish to spread your instruction. It is advisable to **allow at least one week between each set of exercises** (although many people need two). THERE IS NO POINT IN TRYING TO RUSH THROUGH THE EXERCISES, AS A LIFETIME'S BAD HABITS AND THE INABILITY TO RELAX PROPERLY CANNOT BE OVERCOME OVERNIGHT. **Do not be impatient with yourself, and do allow the relaxation to permeate you gradually, for the more slowly you do it the more likely it is that the benefits will become deeply rooted and permanent.**

The small notebook that you have acquired will be invaluable, as the great benefits of learning AT appear slowly and imperceptibly, and it is often by looking back through your notebook that you can appreciate the finesse and delicacy of the technique. It is also an excellent idea to write down your main reasons for wanting to undertake autogenic training, so that if there are any aspects that have not already been dealt with by your regular AT exercises you can use the *positive affirmations* (which you will be taught in lesson 9) to either modify them or help to get rid of them.

SETTING THE SCENE

First and foremost, **always make sure that you are comfortable** before you start your exercises. So see that your bladder and bowels do not need emptying, for there is no way that you can relax if you want to go to the lavatory. It is also advisable to take your shoes off, as during the relaxation you will become aware of how constricting they are. Undo any tight clothing, such as collars, ties, belts and corsets.

Make sure, too, that the room in which you are going to do your mental exercises is comfortably warm, quiet and dimly lit. Although later on you will be able to dissociate completely from all sounds, lights and other external distractions, initially you may become more conscious of them, as the early part of autogenic training is a process of awareness, both internal and external. For unless your mind becomes aware of what is going on within you at various levels, it will be unable to direct its immense healing powers towards dealing with whatever may be the cause of your problem.

How often should you do your exercises? It is best to do them **at least three times a day**, especially initially, so that you get into the routine and discipline of exercising regularly. Do your exercises **once in the morning, once at midday** and **once in the evening or at bedtime.** You may, of course, have to modify this to suit your circumstances. But it is important to stick to this kind of pattern, especially with regard to the midday exercise, as it helps to break the day-long cycle of stress. People with a nine-to-five job, especially if they work in open-plan offices, often say that there is nowhere they can do their exercises. If one is determined enough one can always find somewhere reasonably quiet, such as the lavatory. If you do have to use somewhere like the lavatory, you may not get very much out of your AT initially, especially since none of the usual preliminary preparations, such as lighting and sound, can apply. But don't forget that all you are trying to do at this stage is to discipline yourself into a new routine. Once you have mastered the technique you will be able to get as much out of it in the lavatory as anywhere else!

The time that you take over each set of exercises varies, and will be discussed as we proceed.

REMEMBER THAT THESE FEW MINUTES A DAY THAT YOU GIVE YOURSELF ARE SPECIAL AND THAT YOU DESERVE THEM. SO OFTEN WE FEEL GUILTY ABOUT GIVING OURSELVES THE TIME AND SPACE THAT WE DESERVE. SO DURING THESE MOMENTS REALLY LOVE

YOURSELF, MOLLYCODDLE YOURSELF, AND ENJOY THE SPACE
THAT YOU ARE GIVING YOURSELF. YOU DESERVE IT! GIVE YOURSELF
PERMISSION TO ENJOY YOUR OWN COMPANY AND TO TAKE A WELL
EARNED REST FROM ALL THE PRESSURES AND STRESSES OF EVERY-
DAY LIVING.

YOUR EXERCISE POSITIONS

At each session, you must choose one of the following
positions to do your exercises in. It is best to practise each
position at least once a day. For instance, use the easy chair
position in the morning, the rag-doll position at lunch-time,
and the lying-down position at night before going to sleep,
especially if you want to use your autogenic training TO HELP
YOU TO SLEEP. There are four main positions:

1 The lying-down position

This is the position that most people use at night before going
to sleep, although there is no reason why you should not try it
during the day if you feel that you need a rest or if, for
instance, you suffer from backache. You must be aware,
though, that if you are tired you may fall asleep, even during
the daytime! So until your internal clock has started functioning properly and you can time your AT accurately, set an
alarm clock if you have an important appointment after your
AT session, just to make sure that you do not oversleep!
    Lie on your back with your legs outstretched and slightly
apart, and your feet falling outwards. Your arms should lie by
your sides and your palms facing downwards. You can rest
your down-turned hands on your pelvis, if that feels more
comfortable. Make sure that you are really comfortable. Use
a pillow behind your neck or behind your knees if you need it.
Make sure that your head and neck are straight, that you are
facing straight ahead, and that you are as symmetrical as
possible. If you are covered by bed-clothes, make sure that
they are loose and are not constricting you in any way,
especially over your toes.

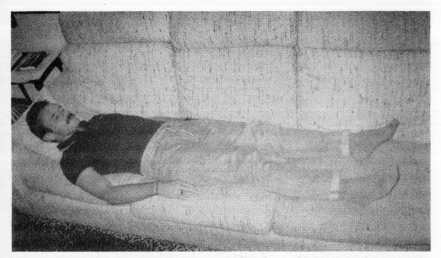

Fig. 1   The lying-down position.

Fig. 2   The easy chair (without arms) position.

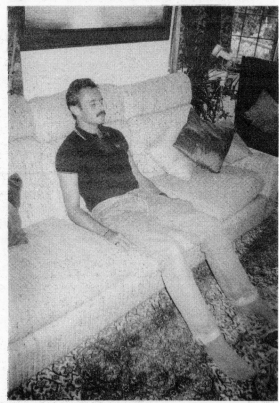

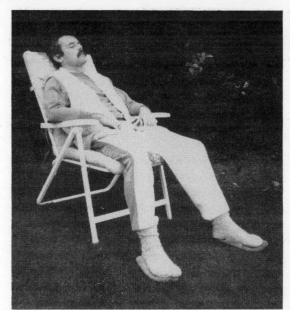

Fig. 3 The easy
chair (with arms)
position.

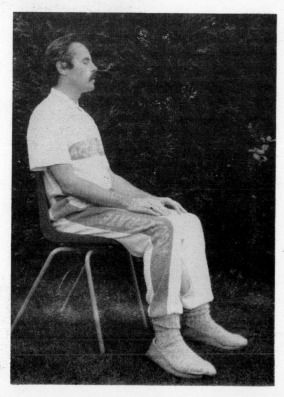

Fig. 4 The meditative
position.

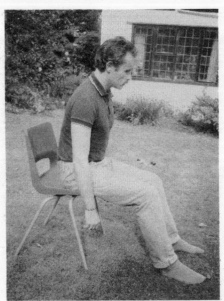

Fig. 5   The rag-doll position, stage 1.

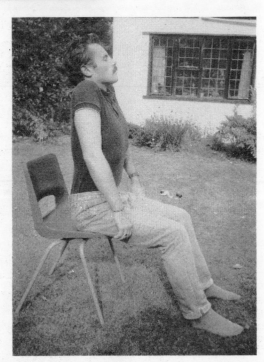

Fig. 6   The rag-doll position, stage 2.

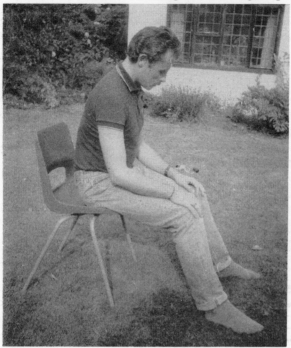

Fig. 7 The rag-doll position, stage 3.

2 The easy chair position

Sit in your favourite easy chair. Your feet must be flat on the floor and about a foot or more apart. Ensure that the angle of your knees is greater than 90 degrees (a right angle), for if it is less it may make your legs go to sleep and become uncomfortable when you relax deeply. Also, ensure that your back and neck are at ease and well supported. Do use a cushion in the small of your back or behind your neck if you need to. Your arms must rest comfortably, either by your sides or on your lap, whichever you prefer. You must ensure that your hands are not clenched, and that your fingers are comfortably straight. If your chair has arms, you may have to rest your own on the arms of the chair, with your fingers stretched out. Now close your eyes.

If your chair has no neck rest, you will have to keep your neck in what we call the neutral position – that is, straight along the line of your back. Do make sure that your head does not flop forwards, especially as you get progressively more relaxed, as that can become uncomfortable and give you a stiff neck, or even give you the feeling that you are rolling forwards or downwards. Although this in itself is of no serious consequence, it can be quite an unpleasant feeling.

3   The meditative position

This is the position that you can adopt in any public situation, such as on trains or buses, or in the doctor's waiting room. Choose an office- or a dining-chair. Sit with your back resting comfortably against the back of the chair, and your neck resting in a straight line with your body, in the neutral position. Place your legs and feet comfortably, with the angle of your knees beyond the right angle, your hands resting on your lap or thighs, and your eyes closed.

4   The rag-doll position

For this position, use an office- or a dining-chair again. Sit forward towards the front of the chair, so that the edge of the seat does not dig into the backs of your legs – if it does, your legs may go to sleep and make you feel uncomfortable. Ensure that your feet are flat on the floor and at least 12 inches apart, with the angle of the knees at more than 90 degrees. This will give you a firm, wide base, so that there is no possibility of your feeling unsafe or unsteady when you relax deeply, especially if you fall asleep in this position. This may seem an impossibility, particularly when you first start doing it and get in touch with all the pains and tensions in your back and neck. But once you have worked through these problems, you will find this position very comfortable and relaxing.

Next, let your arms dangle by your sides, and stretch your back and neck as far up as you can: that is, stretch those big muscles in the back and neck which often go into spasm when one is under stress – hence the frequency of backache and neckache when one is under any form of pressure.

Then, imagine that there is a strip of elastic connecting the top of your head to the ceiling. Allow this elastic to snap, so that your neck and back sink slowly into a gentle curve, with your neck bent slightly forwards. Don't go so far forward that you partially obstruct your windpipe, as that can be very uncomfortable. Then bring your arms up and rest your hands on your lap or thighs. Finally, close your eyes, if you have not already done so.

Although at first you may find that this is not a very comfortable position, especially if you carry a lot of tension in the muscles of your back and neck, as most of us do, it is very important to do it at least once a day. You will find that as time goes on and you manage to offload the tensions, the position will become progressively more comfortable; and if at any time in the future you start carrying more tension in these muscles, you will be able to get rid of the aches and pains by adopting the position more frequently.

You may find that as you relax more and the tension is offloaded from the muscles of the back and neck, you will move either forwards or backwards on your chair. This is perfectly all right, as long as you do not move too much and the position still feels comfortable. If you start bearing weight on your hands and arms, you have moved too far forward and you need to move slightly backwards again. You may find that you have to adjust your position repeatedly, especially at the beginning. Don't worry about that. It is very common and perfectly acceptable, and it certainly does not interfere with your level of relaxation. But if you do not adjust your position to a more comfortable one, then you will be unable to relax. Even people who are very experienced in the technique have to adjust their position from time to time, especially if they start carrying a lot of tension in their backs and necks.

I am now going to introduce three most important procedures – *cancellation* and *scanning* – and *passive concentration*, which is central to the whole concept of autogenic training.

CANCELLATION

The way that we terminate the exercises is usually referred to as *cancellation*. It is particularly important to be able to do it properly later on, when you will go very deep within yourself. Cancelling properly enables you to return to your normal crisp reflexes after you have finished your exercises. Try it several times before you go any further, to ensure that you have got it and can do it properly.

The act of cancelling is a bit like your first yawn and stretch of the day, that you do to wake yourself up. It consists of four steps:

1 **Clench both fists tightly.**
2 **Bend your elbows briskly and stretch your arms right out, either in front of you or sideways.**
3 **Take a deep breath in.**
4 **Open your eyes and breathe out.**

You must be sure to open your eyes last, or the cancellation will not be fully effective, especially if you have gone particularly deep into yourself. If this happens it does not matter very much, so long as you are aware of it and cancel once again. There is nothing to stop you cancelling repeatedly. The important thing is to ensure that you have completely emerged from the AT state.

If you have done your AT in the car it is advisable, before you drive off again, to get out and walk once round the car after you have cancelled. This is particularly important for those who drive long distances on the motorway and use AT to refresh themselves during the journey. Some people feel very self-conscious cancelling like this in public – though I must say I have seen people do far stranger things! Be that as it may, if you want to you can cancel in public places in this less obvious way:

1 Clench your fists tightly.
2 Turn the clenched fists inwards towards each other and push your shoulders back, by arching the spine between your shoulder blades.
3 Take a deep breath in.
4 Open your eyes and breathe out.

If you feel that you are still not fully alert, repeat the cancellation until you feel that you are well out of the AT state.

PASSIVE CONCENTRATION

I mentioned earlier that this is the most important aspect, the mainstay, of the whole autogenic training concept. Although it is very simple in essence, it can at first be quite difficult to achieve. Some people take as long as three or four weeks to achieve total passive concentration. So don't worry or get despondent if you cannot manage it immediately. Eventually you will master it. As I have already said, you may need time: just be patient and gentle with yourself. NOTHING IS EASY WHEN YOU FIRST START, ESPECIALLY WHEN YOU ARE EMBARKING ON A NEW DISCIPLINE IN ORDER TO TRY TO CHANGE THE BAD HABITS AND PATTERNS OF MANY YEARS, EVEN OF A LIFETIME.

Most of our lives we have been taught to concentrate hard and actively. Usually our concentration is aim- and result-oriented: that is, the harder we concentrate and the harder we work, the more likely we are to achieve our goals and to get there more quickly. However, WITH PASSIVE CONCENTRATION WE ARE NOT TRYING TO GET THERE OR, INDEED, TO ACHIEVE ANYTHING. ALL WE ARE TRYING TO DO IS SIT BACK AND WATCH WHAT HAPPENS TO OUR BODIES AND MINDS WHEN WE GO THROUGH THE AUTOGENIC TRAINING FORMULAE (phrases) AND INSTRUCTIONS. This is a very simple concept, but because of our prolonged conditioning in the opposite direction it can at first be quite difficult to achieve.

We so often wonder how we can achieve anything or improve our health and well-being at all if we are not constantly working at it. This is the crux of the matter, and why AT is so different from anything else. We think that we know at a conscious level what is best for us. In fact, IT IS THE INNER WISDOM OF OUR BODIES AND MINDS THAT KNOWS BEST, AND IF WE ALLOW THEM TO COMMUNICATE FREELY AND WITHOUT INTERFERENCE, THEY DO THEIR BEST FOR US. Unfortunately, our conscious interference by means of active concentration usually puts a spanner in the works. With *passive concentration* through the use of autogenic training we are trying to reverse the trend and to allow the healing, regulating and normalising processes of the body to start functioning fully, with a view to improving our health and well-being at all levels and enabling us to fight any disease or disability by drawing upon all our inner, and so far untapped, resources.

SCANNING

Having mastered the positions, learnt how to cancel the exercises and achieve passive concentration, there is just one more procedure that you must learn: you ALWAYS do what we call a *scan* after you have got into position and before you start the exercises proper. The purpose of the scan is twofold: first, to gather yourself together and centre yourself; and second, to get in touch with your body. It is surprising how little contact with or awareness of our bodies we have. We often become aware of them only when some part or other starts to malfunction. In AT we want to connect with our bodies, whatever state they may be in, so that if they are healthy we try to keep them that way, and if they are diseased we try to improve the situation.

Once you are in your chosen position, and have made sure that you are correctly arranged and comfortable, close your eyes. I will explain in a moment exactly how you take your mind to your body bit by bit. It is perfectly all right to move any part as you focus on it. It is important to move and make yourself more comfortable if at any time you become aware that you are uneasy, for it is impossible to relax if you are not comfortable. And remember that there is nothing to stop you scratching yourself if you have an itch, because unless you do, you will be unable to relax.

The important thing is not to dwell on any particular part as you go through your body, especially if you become aware of pain or tension anywhere. Just make a mental note of what you feel in that part and move on to the next. **Once your mind becomes aware of any problems that may be present in any part, it will deal with them for you. You do not have to work hard to reap the benefits of AT. It is most important to enjoy yourself, to enjoy the sessions, and to enjoy the time and the caring, loving space that you are giving yourself; to feel that you well and truly deserve to enrich yourself and your life.** It is only by doing so that you will also be able to enrich the lives of those around you. For the whole thing has a ripple effect: it is like throwing a pebble into the middle of the pond and watching the ripples spread far and wide. The only difference is that in this instance the ripples are those of love, caring, well-being, peace and tranquillity.

This is how you do it:

Take your mind to your feet, starting with the toes. Make sure that you take in both sides of your body simultaneously. (It might be difficult to do that initially. Don't worry; just take your time. It will eventually come to you.) **Then move up your feet to your heels, then to your ankles, calves, shins, thighs, hips and pelvis, stomach, chest, shoulders, upper arms, elbows, forearms, wrists, hands and fingers. Now take your mind to your back, starting with the buttocks, up the big muscles of the back, around the shoulder blades, up the back of the neck, over the scalp, the forehead, around the eyes, the cheeks, and the jaw, which should hang loosely and comfortably.**

If you find that you have difficulty in getting in touch with one or more parts or all of your body – which is reasonably common – you may find it easier if, with eyes closed, you run your hands over the various parts of your body, as indicated above. Once you have done it a few times, you will find that it becomes easier to do it mentally without having to get in touch with your body physically. Another way that makes it easier for some people is to imagine that you are giving yourself a massage as you go through each part of the body. Yet others find it helpful to imagine an enormous paintbrush running all over the various parts of their bodies as they do the scan. You may have to try all these ways until you find the one that you like. And you may discover yet other ways that suit you and your personality. Whatever you choose is perfectly all right, as long as it feels right and comfortable and enables you to get in touch with all of your body.

Most people find that at first they like to go through the scan very slowly, to ensure that they get in touch with every part of their bodies. Don't forget that I am giving only a guideline, and that you can always add other parts omitted here but that you find particularly tense. Once you have mastered the technique, you may find that you want to go through the scan very quickly. The speed with which you do it is really immaterial; the important thing is always to go through the same routine in the same way, and to get in touch with all parts of your body as you go through the scan.

56 *Preliminaries: exercise positions and other essentials*

Having absorbed the above points and mastered the techniques described, you are very nearly ready to proceed with the first exercise. But first, a few last important points.

§10 Before you start

I am going to assume that **you will spend at least one week on each new lesson**, and the instructions are based on this premise. If you are going to spend a longer time on each, you can easily make the necessary adjustments.

There is a great temptation to try to rush through the exercises, if only out of curiosity to see what happens. We are all guilty of this from time to time. *Please* resist the temptation, though, as you will not do yourself any favours if you do rush. As I have already mentioned, it takes time to change, and even more to reverse, the bad habits of a lifetime. Don't be discouraged or despondent, either, if you don't seem to be able to relax or to get much out of the exercises initially. **Be patient, gentle, caring and loving with yourself, and don't get upset or angry or feel guilty about the fact that you may not be doing the exercises properly or achieving very much so far.** We are very good at admonishing and chastising ourselves, but find it hard to take ourselves for what we are and give ourselves permission to take time and to allow the mind to proceed as slowly or as fast as it wants to.

REMEMBER THAT TOTAL RELAXATION OF ANY KIND, INCLUDING THAT DERIVED FROM AUTOGENIC TRAINING, IS AN IMPOSSIBLE TASK, AND NONE OF US, NO MATTER HOW EXPERIENCED, CAN QUITE MANAGE IT! SO DO THE BEST YOU CAN AND ENJOY YOURSELF. Another factor that seems to worry a lot of people at first is that they get distracted by their thoughts and cannot let their minds go blank! This is another point on which AT varies from other forms of relaxation and meditation. For we accept that we *cannot* turn off the computer of the brain and mind and that thoughts are bound to come in and out. We accept these thoughts for what they are, and as soon as we become aware that we are being distracted by them we bring our attention to the task in hand, firmly but gently. Once we become proficient at the exercises, we learn to dissociate ourselves from the intruding thoughts in such a way that they do not interfere with our state of relaxation. They become like fluffy white clouds drifting on the far horizons of our minds.

We discussed in §9 how often you should do your exercises. Obviously, the more often you do them, the more quickly you will be able to get into AT and derive the full benefits. **The more you put into it, the more you will be able to get out of it.** This is a lot more difficult to put into practice than it sounds, and the most difficult point of all is to discipline oneself to do the AT exercises every day. You will find the 'rat factor' (§4) very active, especially in the early stages, and you will discover an enormous number of excuses for not doing your exercises and for postponing them! **Do beware of the 'rat'!** I repeat: do your exercises **at least three times a day**, and preferably **using a different position at each session**. It is best to do them MORNING, NOON and NIGHT.

THREE GOLDEN RULES

Before going any further, please note the THREE GOLDEN RULES that must be observed while you go through the exercises. **This applies to all the exercises throughout the lessons that follow.**

1 **Cancel immediately** if you get in touch with any particularly uncomfortable feelings or sensations.
2 **Cancel immediately** if you start seeing *concrete images*: for instance, if you see a swan swimming over a beautiful calm pond. NEVER dwell on or follow these images, no matter how pleasant they may be. For they can open up a can of worms in the unconscious and make us aware of some unpleasant memory or feeling. When we start doing our AT, we do not particularly want to bring these memories or experiences to the conscious level. If there is anything that needs to be worked through, we would like it worked through slowly and gently at the unconscious level. DON'T FORGET – THE WHOLE CONCEPT OF AT IS BASED ON PASSIVITY AND GENTLENESS.
3 You will use certain set phrases, or formulae, which will

be explained as we go along. **Never** change them, thinking that you know best. They have been chosen after many years of experience and research as being the safest and the most beneficial ones. If you do not heed this warning, you may get yourself into a great deal of trouble. Here are two examples that illustrate this point.

One trainee thought that her symptoms were not in her limbs – which is where we normally start focusing with the heaviness exercises (see pages 62, 69) – but in her brain. So she changed the phrase, despite the usual warning, to 'My brain is heavy'. Needless to say, she ended up with severe and intractable headaches, which fortunately disappeared after further treatment and the use of the correct formulae. The other case involves a man who, because he had always felt too warm, decided to change the formula to 'My arm is cold'. His arm went into an irreversible spasm, and he had to be hypnotised for some time in order to reverse the unwanted changes.

Finally, a word of caution. You may have to modify or even leave out one or more of the lessons that follow if you start having problems with any of them. Please be guided by the instructions in each lesson and what is coming up for you. Do not try and force anything through; not only will that not help you, it can actually be counterproductive and detrimental.

Lesson 1 The short exercise and the heaviness-in-the-limbs exercises

Lesson 1 is divided into three parts and spans one week, assuming that you are spending one week on each lesson. If you have decided that you need longer, spread it out over two weeks.

DAY 1: THE SHORT EXERCISE

Having made a mental note of the golden rules just outlined, you are now ready to proceed with this first exercise.

Although the *short exercise* is very simple, it is a very important one and **has several uses**:

1 It helps to train you to concentrate and to attain and maintain the AT state.
2 It can be practised when you haven't much time.
3 It can be used at times when you feel very emotional or angry, or are in a lot of pain, when it is not usually possible to concentrate sufficiently on the longer exercises.
4 It can be used repeatedly during the day to top up the relaxing effects of the other exercises.

With the short exercise, we concentrate on the **feeling of heaviness in the dominant arm** – the right arm for right-handed people and the left arm for those who are left-handed. The phrase, or formula, that we use is '**My right** (left) **arm is heavy**'. Remember that your arm starts at your shoulder and goes all the way down to the tips of your fingers. So when you repeat the phrase quietly to yourself, connect up with your dominant arm and let your mind travel down the whole length of it. **It is important not to expect anything at all to happen.** All you do is repeat the phrase and sit back and passively observe what may be happening to that arm. **Don't expect it to go heavy – in fact, don't do anything at all.** Just note what is happening.

You may find that your arm actually goes heavy. On the other hand, it may go light or warm, or you may notice pins and needles or some other sensation in it. You may even find that nothing at all happens. That is perfectly all right too. Just note what's happening, and at the end of the exercise record the feelings in your notebook.

Different people have different ways of repeating the formulae to themselves and of connecting to the part to which they are talking. Some like to hear the phrases in their minds; others prefer to see the instructions written in their mind's eye. Both are perfectly acceptable. You must find the way that suits you best and stick with it. However, **it is essential, irrespective of which method you use, that you mentally connect with that part.**

Now, to do the exercise. First, choose your AT position. **Get into it correctly** (see page 45), and make sure that you are comfortable. Next, **do the scan** (see page 54), and then take your mind to your dominant arm. Now **repeat 3 times** the phrase, 'My right (left) arm is heavy' quietly to yourself. Then cancel (see page 51). **Repeat the whole sequence 3 times.** You do not have to scan between cancellations, unless you find that you have become particularly tense again in some part or parts of your body. After the final cancellation, jot down in your notebook the feelings that you have experienced.

This is your first exercise and your introduction to AT, and I would like you to repeat it several times during the next twenty-four hours. The more you manage to do, the better. Simple, isn't it?

SUMMARY OF THE SHORT EXERCISE

Get into your chosen AT position.
Scan.
Take your mind to your dominant arm (right or left).
Repeat 3 times 'My right (left) arm is heavy'.
Do a quick cancel.

Repeat the whole procedure (excluding the scan between cancellations) 3 times.

Homework Do this exercise several times during the first twenty-four hours, and record your experience in your notebook.

Now that you have mastered the short exercise, you can proceed to the first stage of the full exercise which follows.

DAYS 2–4: HEAVINESS IN BOTH ARMS

On days 2, 3 and 4, include both arms. But don't forget to cancel immediately if you get in touch with uncomfortable or unpleasant feelings or sensations, or start seeing images. The exercise for days 2,3 and 4 goes as follows:

Get into an AT position.
Scan.
'My right (left) arm is heavy' – **repeat 3 times**.
'My left (right) arm is heavy' – **repeat 3 times**.
'My arms are heavy' – **repeat 3 times**.
Cancel.

Repeat the whole exercise (excluding the scan between cancellations) **3 times**.

After the final cancellation, write a brief note of your experiences in your notebook.

Homework Repeat the exercise for days 2–4 at least 3 times each day, making sure that you use all three main positions.

DAYS 5–7: HEAVINESS IN BOTH ARMS AND LEGS

On days 5, 6 and 7, include your legs as well. Remember that your leg starts from the hip and goes right down as far as the tips of your toes. So the exercise for the remaining days of the week is as follows:

Get into an AT position.
Scan.
Take your attention to your dominant arm, and become a passive observer of your body as you go through the exercise:

Repeat the following formulae 3 times each:
'My right (left) arm is heavy.'
'My left (right) arm is heavy.'
'My arms are heavy.'
'My right (left) leg is heavy.'
'My left (right) leg is heavy.'
'My legs are heavy.'
'My arms and legs are heavy.'
Cancel.

Repeat this set of exercises 3 times.

After the final cancellation, write up your experiences briefly in your notebook.

NB. When talking to your arms or your legs, you may find it easier to take a broad view of yourself by including in your mind's eye both of your arms as well as your trunk and both your legs, rather than flitting from one side to the other. This makes it a bit easier not only to do the exercise, but also to begin to make yourself feel symmetrical and whole.

What do I do if I experience any feelings that are too strong or uncomfortable?

If you find that the feelings of heaviness, or any other sensations that you may be feeling, are too strong or uncomfortable, you can reduce the intensity either by cutting down the number of repetitions or by adding the word 'slightly' to the formula: for example, 'My right (left) arm is slightly heavy'.

Homework   Repeat this exercise at least 3 times a day during days 5, 6 and 7, using all the main positions and keeping good notes of your experiences.

SUMMARY OF LESSON 1

After you have done all the preliminaries (§9) thoroughly, concentrate on the feeling of heaviness in your various limbs as follows:

Day 1: short exercise

Get into your chosen AT position.
Scan.
Mentally connect with your dominant arm (right or left).
'My right (left) arm is heavy – repeat 3 times.
Cancel.
Repeat the whole procedure (excluding the scan between cancellations) 3 times, provided that it feels pleasant and comfortable, then several times more during the day. Keep brief notes of your experiences.

Days 2–4: full exercise involving both arms

Get into a correct AT position.
Scan.
Mentally connect with your dominant arm once again.
Repeat the following 3 times each:
    'My right (left) arm is heavy.'
    'My left (right) arm is heavy.'
    'My arms are heavy.'
Cancel.
Repeat the whole procedure (excluding the scan between cancellations) 3 times.
Keep brief notes of your experiences.

Repeat this exercise at least 3 times a day, remembering to cancel immediately if you get in touch with images or uncomfortable sensations.

Days 5–7: full exercise involving both arms and legs

Get into an AT position.
Scan.
Mentally connect with your dominant arm once again.
Repeat the following formulae 3 times each:
'My right (left) arm is heavy.'
'My left (right) arm is heavy.'
'My arms are heavy.'
'My right (left) leg is heavy.'
'My left (right) leg is heavy.'

'My legs are heavy.'
'My arms and legs are heavy.'
Cancel.
Repeat the whole procedure (excluding the scan between the cancellations) 3 times.
Keep a concise note of your experiences.

Repeat this exercise at least 3 times a day using a different position each time, and **remember to cancel immediately if you start seeing images or get in touch with uncomfortable or unpleasant sensations**.

Lesson 2 Add the neck-and-shoulders heaviness exercise

During the last week you may have had some difficulty with your concentration, particularly during days 5–7, which introduce quite a long exercise. Don't worry about this. It is a problem which most trainees experience initially, and it will come right in time. Be understanding and patient with yourself. We all demand far too much of ourselves, and expect everything to work immediately. Relaxation does not work like that, though, and if someone tells you that it does, don't believe them! To learn to relax and improve yourself is hard work and time-consuming, but it is well worthwhile in the long run.

You may also have found that your eyelids have been flickering, or you may have had difficulty in keeping them shut. Flickering eyelids are quite common at this stage, and all it means is that your concentration is not quite what it might be. It will settle down in time. Difficulty in keeping your eyes closed is quite significant: it usually indicates that you are not yet ready to let go and relax completely. Respect that. Remember that your mind will only let you go as far as it feels comfortable and safe for you to go, and no further. Our minds have tremendous protective powers and mechanisms, and will not let us go beyond the point that is right for us.

Whenever we start on anything different, particularly when it concerns relaxation, we may experience a strong fear of letting go or losing control, of going over the edge and not being able to come back again. These are perfectly normal and real unconscious, or even conscious, fears and reservations. RESPECT THEM. For your mind will let you go once it has developed enough confidence that you are not going to lose control, and that you will always be in control, even when you are at the deepest levels of relaxation. If you have any particular fears or worries in this context it might be worth your while to write them down or discuss them with a trusted

friend or even a professional counsellor (see Appendix 1) or
therapist, if you feel that that could help you. Often by
expressing the fear or the worry and so externalising it, you
can help to get it out of the unconscious and thus out of
the way, so that it will not go on causing problems in the
future.

The other thing that may have happened during the last
week is that you may have become much more aware of
external distractions such as noise and light, as well as of
internal ones such as tension and aching in areas that you were
totally unaware of previously. This is quite common as well.
For, as I mentioned earlier, the initial week or two is mainly a
process of developing self-awareness and self-realisation; for
until or unless we become aware of what is going on within
and outside us there is no way that we, or our minds, can do
anything about any of it.

As far as external problems and distractions are concerned,
either our minds learn to dissociate from them or, if they are a
particular source of worry and stress, we do something about
them on a conscious level, in order to obviate their detrimental effects on us and on our way of living. As for bodily
tensions and aches and pains, these are the only ways that our
bodies and minds have of telling us where the problems lie.
Do not just dismiss them out of hand: **listen to them** and take
note of them. It is only by acknowledging them that we can
become aware of the possible sources of our difficulties, and
our minds can then concentrate all their healing powers on the
problem areas and help to improve our lot.

You may also have found that during some exercises you
have become a lot more relaxed than in others. In fact, you
may not have become at all relaxed in some of them. This,
too, is quite a common happening. Remember that no two
AT exercises are ever the same, no matter how experienced
you are. How you feel during each exercise will depend to
some extent on what is going on around you as well as inside
you, and how active the 'rat' (§4) may be in that particular
instance. Even if you do not seem to be getting very much
out of some exercises, **do persist with them** and do them
regularly. You will find that things improve, and if there
are any resistances you will be able to work through them in
time.

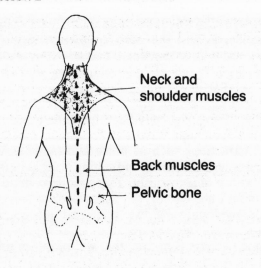

Back view

Fig. 8   The neck and shoulder muscles.

In this lesson we concentrate on the **feeling of heaviness in the muscles of the neck and shoulders**. This is a particularly important area, as most of us carry an enormous amount of tension and repressed emotions and feelings here. So it is well worthwhile spending a little time getting familiar with the area and with the extent of the muscles involved.

I will start with a short description of the neck and shoulder muscles, just in case you are not familiar with them. They occupy quite a large expanse, and since they are situated behind us and we do not normally pay much attention to them, it can at first be quite difficult to get in touch with them. It can be made quite a lot easier, though, if you run your hands over the area where the muscles are, or it may be more effective if you get someone else to do it for you. You will see from figure 8 that the back muscles are two large and powerful structures resembling a series of cords, that extend the full length of the spine on either side of the bony prominences (the vertebrae) that you can feel if you pass your fingers over it, starting from the buttocks and ending at the base of the skull. The large sheet of flattish neck muscles overlies the back muscles at the top of the spine. They start at the base of the skull and extend downwards and outwards over the shoulders, forming a roughly triangular shape as far as the middle of the back. As you can see, the neck and shoulder muscles are pretty large and powerful, so it is hardly surprising that when they go into spasm or become tense we end up with severe neckache, headache or backache, or all three! Tension in this area can often lead to attacks of migraine.

THE STANDARD (FULL) NECK-AND-SHOULDERS HEAVINESS EXERCISE

The phrase that we use here is '**My neck and shoulders are heavy**'. Afterwards we add '**I am at peace**'. When we say the first phrase we try to connect mentally with the muscles of the neck and shoulders. You may find it difficult at first to get in touch with them. Don't worry: it will come in time, especially if at the same time you or someone else touches the area. You may be more likely to get in touch with your neck and shoulders in the rag-doll position (page 50) where your neck is unsupported, rather than in any of the other positions, although if you are particularly tense in that area you may get in touch with it in other positions as well. In that case you may find that your neck becomes more painful for a while, especially during the exercise. This is perfectly in order. It is not that the exercise is making your neck more painful; you are just getting in touch with the large amount of tension that you are carrying in that area. In time the tension will work through, and the pain and discomfort with it.

When you mention the phrase 'I am at peace', try to keep your mind blank, but if a peaceful image occurs to you, that's all right. Cancel immediately, though, if the image changes to something that is not peaceful, or if you get an unpeaceful or unpleasant image right from the beginning. Just try again later.

At this point we summarise the first lesson's heaviness-in-the-limbs exercise and add this week's phrases at the end of it, so that the new full formula will be as follows:

'My right (left) arm is heavy' – **say this once.**
'My arms and legs are heavy' – **repeat 3 times.**

'My neck and shoulders are heavy' – **repeat 3 times.**
'I am at peace' – **repeat 3 times.**

From now on we say 'My right (left) arm is heavy' only once, and this is known as the *trigger formula*. Although we normally perform only the above version of the heaviness-in-the-limbs exercise at this stage, there is no reason why you should not go through the full version that you learned in lesson 1, if you so wish. But most people find that it is too long, and that they get as much out of the exercise by using the shortened version.

So your exercise for the next week is as follows:

Get into a correct AT position.
Scan.
Mentally connect with your dominant arm (right or left), and become a passive observer of yourself and see what happens as you go through the new formula:
'My right (left) arm is heavy' – **say this once.**
'My arms and legs are heavy' – **repeat 3 times.**
'My neck and shoulders are heavy' – **repeat 3 times.**
'I am at peace' – **repeat 3 times.**
Cancel.

Repeat this procedure **3 times** (excluding the scan in between the cancellations).

Repeat the whole exercise **at least 3 times a day**, using different positions for each session.

THE PARTIAL NECK AND SHOULDERS EXERCISE

Apart from forming part of the standard exercise, the *neck and shoulders exercise* can also be used as what we call a *partial exercise*. For this, you only need to repeat the phrase 'My neck and shoulders are heavy' over and over again – and the more you repeat it, the better!

To use 'My neck and shoulders are heavy' as a partial exercise:

Do not take your mind to your neck and shoulders.
Do not close your eyes.

Do not get into an AT position.
Do not add the phrase 'I am at peace'.

Just repeat 'My neck and shoulders are heavy' over and over, quietly to yourself. It is so easy to forget to do this, so in order to remind yourself you can GET YOURSELF SOME OF THOSE SMALL COLOURED STICKY DOTS AND PUT THEM IN STRATEGIC PLACES, SO that every time you see one, or see something of the same colour, it reminds you to repeat the phrase 'my neck and shoulders are heavy'. For the partial exercise, you need to say it at least 70 to 100 times a day. We often tend to choose blue for this purpose, as blue has been found to be relaxing. But what matters is that whenever you see your chosen colour it reminds you to do your exercises.

You may find that at first you do not get very much out of this partial exercise. But if you persevere you will find that IN TIME IT WILL BECOME A VERY EFFECTIVE EXERCISE FOR REDUCING YOUR STRESS LEVEL, PARTICULARLY MUSCULAR TENSIONS, IN SITUATIONS WHERE YOU CANNOT NORMALLY DO YOUR STANDARD AT EXERCISES – THAT IS, YOUR FULL EXERCISES – SUCH AS WHILE DRIVING, WALKING OR IN THE MIDDLE OF BUSY MEETINGS. You can also use this exercise when you are particularly angry or distressed, in order to try to control your emotions and deal with the situation in a calmer and more rational way.

SUMMARY OF LESSON 2

The standard exercise (using 'My neck and shoulders are heavy' and 'I am at peace')

Get into a correct AT position.
Scan.
Get mentally in touch with your dominant arm:
'My right (left) arm is heavy' – say it once.
'My arms and legs are heavy' – repeat 3 times.
'My neck and shoulders are heavy' – repeat 3 times.
'I am at peace' – repeat 3 times.
Cancel.

Repeat the above exercise (excluding the scan in between the cancellations) 3 times. Keep a note of your experiences in your notebook.

The partial exercise
Use 'My neck and shoulders are heavy' as a partial exercise in which you constantly repeat the phrase to yourself, using the blue labels (or whatever colour you have chosen) to remind you to do it at least 70 to 100 times a day.

Homework   Use the full (standard) exercise, repeating each set 3 times before the final cancellation, at least 3 times a day and using all the main positions. Use the partial exercise repeatedly throughout the day, initially to just get into the habit, and then use it to top up the effects of the full exercise in between times.

Use the *short exercise*, 'My right (left) arm is heavy', as much as possible, when you get a few moments, in order to enhance and reinforce the effects of the full exercise. Don't forget about its other uses (lesson 1).

Lesson 3   Add the warmth-in-the-limbs exercise

I hope you have been doing your exercises regularly and using the neck and shoulders partial exercise on numerous occasions. As I mentioned in lesson 2, the more you use it, the more you will get out of it in the long run.

People often say at this stage that they want to do the exercises without cancelling in between the sets. 'I am just getting into it, and I have to cancel!' is a common cry. Later, we will start to prolong the exercises, and to go much deeper. But at this stage we do not want to go too deep, for if we did, any unresolved problems, emotions or memories might flood into the conscious from the unconscious. We might well find this too uncomfortable or even too difficult to deal with, particularly if it happened in one great rush. What we want to do is allow these unresolved problems to work through gently and slowly, without necessarily coming into the conscious. So go slowly, gently and patiently, and it will pay in the long term.

In this lesson we start concentrating on the feeling of warmth in the limbs. As I said earlier, these exercises follow the normal sequence of physiological changes that occur in the body when we relax. As the muscles relax, so the blood vessels open and the circulation to any given part increases; hence we feel warmth in that part. Some of you may have already noticed this phenomenon while doing the previous exercises, especially if you have become particularly relaxed from time to time. Furthermore, as the bloodflow to the various parts of the body increases, you may become aware of throbbing or pulsing in those parts. This is a perfectly normal part of the process of relaxation, though it may be quite alarming when you become aware of pulsations or heartbeats for the first time.

Remember that although in this exercise you concentrate on the feeling of warmth, you will not necessarily get that sensation, for like any other feeling that we may talk about here, it will not be experienced by everyone: up to 30–40 per cent of trainees do not get one or more of the sensations that they are focusing on. This is perfectly normal and acceptable, and it does not mean that your AT is not going to work for you. The end result – achieving relaxation – is exactly the same, irrespective of whether or not you get the sensations that you focus on *en route*. In fact, by the time you are very deeply relaxed you may not get any sensations at all; you may be able to dissociate altogether from physical sensations, which is fine, particularly if you are suffering from a condition characterised by a lot of pain, discomfort or distress. To be able to dissociate from these symptoms even for a short while during your AT state will help you to cope with them much more effectively when you come out of that state.

You may have already noticed that you are twitching a lot in the muscles of your limbs. This often happens if you carry a lot of tension there: the twitching is part of your body de-stressing itself. If that is the case, you may find it helpful to do the *motor-loosening exercise* (page 90) before your scheduled AT exercise.

The most important thing is to passively observe what sort of feelings or sensations you are getting, if any. Even while concentrating on the feeling of warmth in your limbs you may experience a feeling of coldness, especially if your surroundings are not particularly warm or if you are carrying a lot of negative feelings, emotions or memories at the limb level, which is the most superficial at which we carry our bundle of tension. Some of you may also become more acutely aware of emotions such as anxiety or anger. This may present itself as an overt sensation of the emotion or as a less obvious manifestation of it, such as difficulty in concentrating, irritability, increasing tensions in the neck or other muscle groups, or increasing aches and pains in different parts, especially during AT. You may find that your muscles twitch more than usual during AT, or during the night while you are asleep. All these symptoms mean is that you are getting in touch with unresolved or repressed past stress or emotion. This is quite common; a great many people hit a turbulent patch during the third to fifth weeks of the exercises.

I'll give you an example here, which may be useful in

indicating what might happen while you are doing AT during your weeks of training. Imagine that you are crossing the Channel from England to France. When you first leave port, the waters are smooth and calm. This is the equivalent of the first part of your AT sessions. When you reach the middle of the Channel, the water becomes quite turbulent; this is the middle part of your AT exercises (usually between the third and fifth weeks). The waters get smooth and peaceful again once you are approaching the French coast – the terminal part of the exercises. This does not necessarily mean that everybody will follow the same pattern, or that if your pattern is different from this, either AT is not working for you or you are not doing it properly!

Fortunately we are all different, and we all carry with us different luggage at different stages of incompleteness. Therefore what reactions – sometimes known as *discharges* – we get when we do AT is to a large degree dependent on the amount of unresolved or unfinished business that we may have within us, to what extent we are in touch with that unfinished business, and how far on the road to self-discovery and improvement we are. Whether you get a lot of these reactions or none at all is not really relevant. The important thing, if you get in touch with any such unresolved feelings or emotions, is to deal with them through the *offloading exercises* which I describe in lesson 5.

The other thing that you may get in touch with is the pain or discomfort of a previous injury or operation, particularly if you have not yet dealt with the emotional pain of it. Fortunately we usually work through the traumas of our lives at the time that they occur, and it is only occasionally that, for one reason or another, this may not have happened. It may then cause problems at a later stage in our lives. If you get in touch with such unresolved traumas, the experience of the pain may be momentary or it may occur in a few AT sessions before it spontaneously resolves itself and leaves you. It is important to verbalise or externalise any memories or thoughts that may be associated with these feelings, by writing them down or saying them out loud, or by using the *offloading exercises* (lesson 5). Once you give voice to them, then they are extracted from your mind and do not go on causing you trouble in the future.

However, if you find that a particularly uncomfortable sensation or pain, especially if it also occurs outside your AT sessions, fails to settle down quickly, particularly after using the offloading techniques described in lesson 5, you should consult your doctor, in order to ensure that there is no physical problem underlying the pain or discomfort that you are experiencing.

The introduction to the warmth exercise is quite similar to that for the heaviness exercise of lesson 1, insofar as we go through each limb spearately. We introduce this exercise between the heaviness exercise of lesson 1 and 'My neck and shoulders are heavy', lesson 2, which from now on will always come at the end of the full exercise: a bit like a bookend, so that whenever we get to that phrase we will know that we are getting towards the end of that set of exercises.

DAYS 1–3: THE WARMTH EXERCISE IN THE ARMS

The full exercise for the first three days is as follows:

Get into a correct AT position.
Scan.
Get in touch with your dominant arm (right or left), then just become a passive observer of your body and see what happens as you go through the following exercises:
'My right (left) arm is heavy' – **once.**
'My arms and legs are heavy' – **3 times.**
'My right (left) arm is warm' – **3 times.**
'My left (right) arm is warm' – **3 times.**
'My arms are warm' – **3 times.**
'My neck and shoulders are heavy' – **3 times.**
'I am at peace' – **3 times.**
Cancel.

Repeat this exercise **3 times**, at least 3 times a day, **provided that you do not have unpleasant, uncomfortable or very strong sensations. If you do, either reduce the number of repetitions or introduce the phrase 'slightly warm' into the exercise instead of 'warm'.** You may even have to leave the warmth exercise out altogether for a day or two if the feelings are very strong, and reintroduce it slowly by saying it once to begin with and then gradually increasing the number of repetitions. Make brief but pertinent notes about your experiences in your notebook.

DAYS 4–7: THE WARMTH EXERCISE IN THE ARMS AND LEGS

In days 4–7, introduce warmth into the legs as well, taking into account the warning in the paragraph above. So the full formula for the rest of the days of the week is as follows:

Get into a comfortable AT position.
Scan.
Start by concentrating on your dominant arm, and just become a passive observer of your body and see what happens as we go through the formula:
'My right (left) arm is heavy' – **once.**
'My arms and legs are heavy' – **3 times.**
'My right (left) arm is warm' – **3 times.**
'My left (right) arm is warm' – **3 times.**
'My arms are warm' – **3 times.**
'My right (left) leg is warm' – **3 times.**
'My left (right) leg is warm' – **3 times.**
'My legs are warm' – **3 times.**
'My arms and legs are warm' – **3 times.**
'My neck and shoulders are heavy' – **3 times.**
'I am at peace' – **3 times.**
Cancel.

Repeat this exercise (excluding the scan in between the cancellations) **3 times**, at least 3 times a day in the three main positions, **unless you have very strong reactions**, in which case either reduce the repetitions or introduce the word 'slightly', as mentioned above. Keep good and relevant notes.

SUMMARY OF LESSON 3 (AND HOMEWORK)

Provided that there are no major problems, as outlined above, proceed as follows:

Days 1–3
Get into an AT position.
Scan.
'My right (left) arm is heavy' – once.
'My arms and legs are heavy' – 3 times.
'My right (left) arm is warm' – 3 times.
'My left (right) arm is warm' – 3 times.
'My arms are warm' – 3 times.
'My neck and shoulders are heavy' – 3 times.
'I am at peace' – 3 times.
Cancel.
Repeat the whole procedure 3 times, at least 3 times a day, using the different positions. Keep notes of your experiences.

Days 4–7
Get into an AT position.
Scan.
'My right (left) arm is heavy' – once.
'My arms and legs are heavy' – 3 times.
'My right (left) arm is warm' – 3 times.
'My left (right) arm is warm' – 3 times.
'My arms are warm' – 3 times.
'My right (left) leg is warm' – 3 times.
'My left (right) leg is warm' – 3 times.
'My legs are warm' – 3 times.
'My arms and legs are warm' – 3 times.
'My neck and shoulders are heavy' – 3 times.
'I am at peace' – 3 times.
Cancel.
Repeat the whole procedure 3 times, at least 3 times a day, using different positions. Keep a note of your experiences.

Using the sticky blue dots (or anything of your chosen colour) as a reminder, do 'My neck and shoulders are heavy' as a *partial exercise*, repeating it at least 70 times a day.

Use the *short exercise* (lesson 1) to top up your relaxation during the day between doing the full standard exercises.

Lesson 4   Add the heartbeat exercise

Bear in mind that, as I have already stressed, it is quite common for trainees to get in touch with certain feelings or emotions that need attention, and that it is important to deal with them by doing one or more of the *offloading exercises* discussed in lesson 5. **So it is very important that you study this chapter and the next one together, and that you use them together, as they are integral parts of each other.**

One of the main presenting symptoms when you, the trainee, are getting in touch with your emotions is loss or deterioration of concentration during the exercises, although you were probably concentrating adequately until then. Beware of the 'rat' (§4) and of the mischievous havoc that it may be playing with your exercises as well, as overactivity in that department can also be a result of your getting in touch with some unresolved or unworked-through feelings or emotions.

By now some of you may be feeling worse than when you started, and may consequently be wondering why on earth you are doing this autogenic training! Don't worry or get despondent, if this is what is happening. For some people, getting in touch with and getting rid of those unwanted emotions may be the most important thing to do at this stage. If this includes you, the relaxation may at this point be secondary. But it will definitely follow, once you have ironed out your problems. It may be hard work and time-consuming, though. So be patient and gentle with yourself, and remember that all good things come to those who take their time in moving towards their goal.

In this lesson we introduce the phrase **'My heartbeat is calm and regular'**. Before we talk about that, though, it is important to know where your heart is actually situated. It is surprising how many people have no idea where it is! The normal heart is usually about the size of a fist. It is situated in the lower part of the chest, with its right edge along the right side of the sternum (breast bone) and its tip, in men, about level with the nipple, and in women, at a corresponding point.

Some of you will have already felt the sensation of pulsing or heartbeat during your warmth exercise, so you know the rate that you might expect. For those of you who have not experienced it yet, you can do so by taking your pulse and observing the rate. You can take your pulse at your wrist, temple, neck or heart region. However, if you cannot or do not want to do it, it doesn't really matter. You may become aware of it when you do your exercises, anyway. However, as I mentioned earlier, whether you get any sensation or not does not really matter; what is far more important is to remember that, whether or not you feel any, they will not interfere with the depth of your relaxation.

The cardiac, or heart, level that we are now entering is quite a deep one. This means that if there are any repressed feelings, emotions or memories at this level, you can become aware of them or their physical manifestations at this stage. One of the first things that may happen when you feel your heartbeat for the first time is that you may feel anxious, uncomfortable or uneasy. It may be a shock to feel your pulse for the first time. These feelings are perfectly normal, especially if, as mentioned earlier, you have a lot of unresolved feelings, especially to do with losses of all kinds, including loss of consciousness or even death. This may be particularly the case if you have a fear of dying of a heart attack, or have relations or friends who have had one. You may find, once you have worked through the unresolved or repressed problems, that your awareness of the sensation of your heartbeat is quite reassuring; it is comforting to know that your heart is beating regularly and normally, and to be in touch with its normal functions when it is healthy, not diseased. HOWEVER, FOR SOME OF YOU THIS INITIAL AWARENESS MAY BE TOO UNCOMFORTABLE. IF THIS IS THE CASE, IT MAY BE WORTHWHILE EITHER REDUCING THE NUMBER OF REPETITIONS OR LEAVING OUT ALTOGETHER FOR A WHILE THIS LESSON'S PHRASE, **'My heartbeat is calm and regular'.** Then you can reintroduce it slowly and gently by first of all just repeating it once in one exercise, and then slowly increasing the number of repetitions.

The awareness of uncomfortable sensations may be particularly noticeable in those who have recently had a heart attack and in those who are particularly worried about or afraid of dying. This fear may be at an unconscious level, of course, and the trainee may not be consciously aware of it at all. It is important to realise that the fear of dying is universal. The only difference is that some of us have become aware of it and faced it and worked through the fear and anxiety, and some of us have not, becoming aware of it only now. Whether or not this is your problem, it is important to write down whatever feelings, emotions or memories you may become aware of at this stage. You will probably find that by doing this you will clarify in your own mind the main sources of your anxieties, and are thus able to deal with them constructively; or your externalising of the problem or fear in this way will make it leave you and disappear into thin air. When that happens, you will find that the same problem will not trouble you again. You can, of course, use the *offloading exercises* described in the next lesson in order to deal with the sensations that you have got in touch with.

Despite having done this, if you still find that you become aware of certain strong emotions such as anger, sadness and frustration, then you are well advised to go straight on to lesson 5, which deals with emotions, and offload those feelings using one or more of the exercises described there. If you find that they do not adequately deal with your problems, then this suggests that you have much deeper problems than you originally thought you had, and that you may require the help of other professionals, such as a counsellor, a co-counsellor (see Appendix), a psychotherapist or other health care specialist, depending on what is available and what suits you and your personality.

NB. If your symptoms or the sensations that you are experiencing are really severe, and none of the above suggestions helps immediately, then it is highly advisable that you discontinue your AT exercises and come back to them after you have worked through whatever may be the cause of your problems and severe reactions. You may require counselling or some form of psychotherapy (see p. 297) to help you work through your underlying problems.

As you learn any new exercise you may find that the previous ones become more effective. This is quite common, for as you concentrate on the new exercise you become truly passive about the previous ones, and so they start to become more powerful.

The phrase that we use in this exercise, 'My heartbeat is calm and regular', is introduced, as with lesson 3's phrases, before the neck and shoulders exercise. While we say lesson 4's phrase, we take our minds to the area where the heart is situated. It is important to watch the rest of your body as well, though, and see if you can actually feel the pulse anywhere else. Sometimes you may only feel it in a hand or a foot, and for only a short while; and even in this one exercise it may flit from one part of the body to another. This is perfectly normal. I am sure that you realise that with every heartbeat the whole of your body pulsates. We may only become aware of the pulsations at a few points in the body during this exercise. **These points (if felt) may be anywhere at all.**

At this stage we amalgamate the heaviness and warmth exercises (lessons 1–3) into one, so that the full formula for the next week will be as follows:

'My right (left) arm is heavy' **– once.**
'My arms and legs are heavy and warm' **– 3 times.**
'My heartbeat is calm and regular' **– 3 times.**
'My neck and shoulders are heavy' **– 3 times.**
'I am at peace' **– 3 times.**

If you have not experienced any major problems and have been managing to relax without any troublesome 'discharges', sensations or emotions, you can now start prolonging the exercises by NOT CANCELLING BETWEEN THE DIFFERENT SETS. It is advisable to start this process slowly, first adding five minutes and gradually building up to an extra twenty. You will find that your concentration will start to wander if you prolong the exercises too soon.

The other important thing at this stage is to enjoy your sessions and not be too dogmatic or regimental about the number of times that you repeat each phrase. So long as you repeat them roughly 3 times, it is perfectly all right. You may find that you will repeat one phrase twice, the next one 4 times and the one after that 3 times. It really does not matter, so long as you go through the exercises in the same suggested sequence. The way to get the maximum benefit from the exercises and to become truly passive about them is to allow the formulae to float gently from one to the next. If you manage to do this you will find that you will start getting much deeper, much more quickly. You may also find that you get especially deep in a particular part of the exercise, and you may want to linger there even though you are only in the first or second set. That is perfectly acceptable too, but the important thing is to complete the exercise by going as far as 'I am at peace' before cancelling. In order to clarify this a bit more, I will give you an example of what I mean.

Let's assume that you want to do your AT for fifteen minutes, but by the time you get to the heartbeat exercise in the first set you are deeply relaxed. You can stay there and enjoy it, provided that your concentration does not wander. You can do this and stay in the relaxed state either by repeating the relevant phrase over and over again or, if your mind is silent, by allowing it to stay silent. Once you feel that the time is up and you want to finish your AT, go on to the neck and shoulders exercise, complete it with 'I am at peace', and then cancel.

Your exercises for the next week, introducing the heartbeat exercise, are as follows:

Get into an AT position.
Scan.
Take your attention to your dominant arm (right or left), then just become a passive observer of your body and see what happens as you go through the formulae.
'My dominant arm (right or left) is heavy' **– once.**
'My arms and legs are heavy and warm' **– 3 times.**
'My heartbeat is calm and regular' **– 3 times.**
'My neck and shoulders are heavy' **– 3 times.**
'I am at peace' **– 3 times.**
Repeat the whole procedure 3 or 4 times.
Cancel.

Repeat the exercises at least 3 times a day, using different AT positions. Keep notes of your experiences after each session.

If you get any strong, uncomfortable feelings or emotions or start seeing concrete images, **cancel immediately** and try the exercises later. (See page 92 for alternative procedures.)

HOMEWORK

Do your AT exercises as indicated above at least 3 times a day, using different positions.

Repeat the partial exercise, 'My neck and shoulders are heavy', as many times and in as many places as possible.

Try as many of the offloading exercises (lesson 5) as possible in order to get a feel of what they are like.

Don't forget to use the *short exercise*, 'My right (left) arm is heavy', whenever you have a few minutes to spare, in order to top up the standard exercises.

Lesson 5   The offloading exercises

The problem with a lot of us, as I have already suggested, is that we do not allow ourselves to get in touch with either our 'positive' emotions, such as love, joy and laughter, or our 'negative' ones such as anger, rage and sadness; and even if we do get in touch with them, we do not allow ourselves the 'luxury' of expressing them, especially in British society where a blank expression in the face of even the most distressing feelings or pain is often considered a virtue. We are all familiar with the stiff upper lip syndrome! So a great many of us repress these vital sensations, and by so doing we not only store up trouble as far as our future health is concerned, but we also live in a world bleaker than it need be, which lacks the expression and exhibition of emotions and feelings.

We have already touched on the possible effects of repressing the so-called 'negative' emotions in §1. It has been shown conclusively that repressing or failing to deal adequately with emotions such as anger, rage, grief, frustration and anxiety can make us more susceptible to all sorts of diseases, ranging from the simple migraine to cancer. Furthermore, it has been shown that if we accept the diagnosis of serious disease blandly and without either feeling or demonstrating powerful emotions, then the deterioration of our condition and the spread of the disease proceed much faster. IT IS THEREFORE EXTREMELY IMPORTANT THAT WE BECOME AWARE OF AND GET IN TOUCH WITH OUR DEEPER FEELINGS AND EMOTIONS, AND THEN LEARN TECHNIQUES OF GETTING RID OF THEM. For by discharging them successfully we can convert their tremendous negative power into equally strong positive energy, which we can utilise in trying to overcome disease or disability.

It must not be forgotten that 'positive emotions' such as fun and laughter, as well as the expression of creativity in all its forms and manifestations, can all have very beneficial effects in both the maintenance of health and the overcoming of disease, once the state of illness has unfortunately become established.

What the term *offloading* means is that the individual learns to externalise all these normal, natural emotions that we can all feel and get in touch with. These particular exercises constitute an essential part of the whole autogenic training process. By learning to deal with these 'negative' emotions we manage to get rid of them and so avoid storing up trouble for the future.

I cannot stress too often how important it is that you **try one or more of these exercises whenever you get in touch with such emotions,** whether or not they have anything to do with your current AT exercises. And it is even more important to **do them if you get in touch with unresolved feelings and emotions or experience certain physical sensations** (see p. 92) **during your AT exercises.** For if you do not do them, and if you try to re-bury or ignore the feelings, you may well find that it will take you a lot longer to get into deeper states or you may not get there at all, and your AT will suffer accordingly. You may also find that you are not able to get into your AT exercises properly and start losing concentration, although you seemed to be doing well up till now and getting into quite deep states.

No harm will come to you if you do not, or cannot, do these offloading exercises. The choice is obviously yours, as you are the best judge of your feelings and repressed memories and of how best to deal with them. *All* that I ask is that you give them a try, and if you do not derive any benefits, then leave them out. I can assure you, though, that once you have tried them and broken through the inhibitions, the self-consciousness and the resistances that are initially associated with doing some of them, you will find them a great help. So de-stress yourself, and benefit from the full healing powers of the technique. I personally have found them of great benefit, and at times they have been the saviours of my sanity! I do them at least once a day, but sometimes more, depending on what sort of a day I am having. Obviously I don't do all of them each time, because that would be both exhausting and time-consuming. I choose the exercise which seems to be most appropriate to my mood or feelings at the time. But do remember that although you may be vaguely aware of how you feel, and so try an exercise that seems appropriate, you may find that that exercise leads into another, which may in fact be more appropriate for you at that moment. You may also find that there is a quick fluctuation between various exercises. That is perfectly all right. Start with one, and allow your mind to take over and offload what it wants to.

We conveniently classify emotions into categories, but it is important to remember that our feelings and emotions are like a ball of tangled wool deep within us, and we may not be certain which emotion predominates. Just pull one end and watch freely and passively what is unravelled – that is to say, start with one exercise and allow it to go any way it wants to.

Since these exercises are helpful in dealing not only with the emotions of the moment but also with any backlog of repressed emotions and feelings, you can do them, often to good effect, 'from cold': in other words, try one or more of them when you are not feeling anything in particular, and see if anything comes up. Sometimes it will, and sometimes nothing much seems to happen. At least by trying the exercises you get good at doing them, and practice makes perfect.

Some people may find that they have a lot of repressed emotions that they need to work through, but find it difficult, or even impossible, to deal with the exercises described here. If this applies to you, it is imperative that you seek further help in the way of counselling, co-counselling, individual or group therapy, or any of a whole variety of other therapeutic techniques that may be available (see p. 297). **Remember that AT is not a panacea for everything and everyone, and some individuals need extra help depending on what they have stored up over the years.** Those of you who do have difficulty with these exercises may find other ways (discussed later in this lesson) of dealing with your feelings, such as playing a musical instrument or writing down your thoughts and feelings as soon as they surface.

Some people find that while they are doing AT they dream more, and that their dreams become a lot more vivid and memorable. If this happens to you, it is important to jot the details down as soon as you wake up, so that you will not forget them. One important thing to bear in mind is that most of what you see in your dreams or remember about them is in a symbolic language, and that the subject of a dream may have no relevance to the real-life situation that it portrays. What is far more important is to realise what each of those symbols means to you, and what thoughts, emotions and feelings are associated with the dream. Often it is these that can give an indication of what underlying problems there may be, that you may want to deal with. You may also find that just by jotting all these things down you are able to deal with a lot of your inner unresolved conflicts and emotions. If you are particularly interested in interpreting your dreams, see the Further Reading list for a useful reference.

The offloading exercises are classified under specific headings. But it is important to realise, as I have already mentioned, that all the emotions are interlinked and that one may easily lead into another. This is perfectly normal and acceptable. Just give it a go and try some of them, and see what happens.

One of the difficulties with many of the exercises that require the offloading of noise is that most of us live in a home where noise may disturb others. This can be a major cause of resistance to doing the exercises. But there are ways of overcoming this problem, and these will be discussed more fully later in this lesson. You can always do them in the shower while the water is running, under a duvet or blanket, or in your car while it is parked somewhere quiet where you are unlikely to be disturbed. And you can have the radio or television on loudly enough to mask some of the noise.

EXERCISES FOR OFFLOADING MUSCLE TENSION AND FRUSTRATION

Remember that you may have to modify some of the following exercises if you are suffering from any physical disease or disability which makes it difficult or impossible to perform them as indicated below. If you are determined enough, I am sure that you will find a way of doing them that fits your situation.

The screaming exercise

This is one of the simplest exercises to perform in order to offload feelings of frustration, anger, and so on. You know – when you get to a screaming pitch and don't know what to do with yourself? Or you just feel awful and don't know what is the matter? Well, now you can do something about those feelings. Do the *screaming exercise*.

How do I do it?

The easiest thing is to **take a deep breath in and scream from the pit of your stomach**, having first of all made sure that you are not in public! Most people find that they are unable to do this freely because they fear being overheard by neighbours or other members of the family. If this is your problem, don't imagine that you can use it as an excuse for not doing the exercise! There is another way of doing it which will bypass these objections.

Sit down and put a large soft pillow on your lap. Take your glasses off if you wear them. (Contact lenses can be left in.) Take a deep breath in, and then scream as loudly as you can from the pit of your stomach, holding the cushion to your face as you do so. Repeat this process several times over, until you feel emptied! Then sit for a few moments and rest, and observe how much better you feel for having vented all those pent-up feelings. It may take you a little while to do this exercise properly, as some people have initial difficulty in screaming from the pit of the stomach. It does you no great harm if you don't do it. The only thing that it may do is give you a temporary sore throat or hoarse voice – but you may find that well worth the sense of release that you feel!

You can do the screaming exercise any time. I always have a cushion in my consulting room, which I use freely whenever I find that things are getting on top of me – as the working life of a general practitioner can be extremely frustrating.

The tantrum exercise

This is another nice easy one that can offload an enormous amount of physical and emotional tension and frustration.

How do I do it?

Lie on your back on a bed, sofa or other soft surface – you can
hurt yourself if you try to do it on a hard surface such as the
floor. Then **pretend to be a child having a tantrum! Beat your
arms and legs rapidly against the bed and scream at the same
time, or make any other noises that naturally want to escape
from you.** Do it for as long as it feels comfortable. Then rest
for a few minutes by lying still. You will find this exercise
enormously releasing. It is one of my own personal
favourites. Once you have been through the whole gamut of
exercises, undoubtedly you will find your own favourites too.

The motor-loosening exercise

This exercise is very useful for offloading excessive amounts
of muscle tension. The problem may present itself as a
straightforward stiffness or tension in the muscles during
everyday activities, as excessive twitches or trembling, or as
restlessness and a constant desire to move during AT exercises. It may also be a useful exercise to try if you twitch a lot
in the night and if your limbs keep jumping, thereby disturb-
ing both your sleep and, perhaps, that of a partner. It can also
be a useful way of offloading the tension and frustration which
may be associated with not having an adequate sexual outlet.

IT IS ALSO QUITE A USEFUL EXERCISE TO DO BEFORE DOING YOUR
AT if you suffer from any of the above problems, or if you find
that you keep losing concentration soon after starting to do
your AT.

How do I do it?

Stand up and close your eyes.
Do a quick upward scan, starting at your feet, then proceeding
to your calves and shins, thighs, hips, stomach, chest, arms,
back, neck, scalp and face.
Make a mental note of any parts that may be especially tense.
Open your eyes.
**Gently move and shake all the parts of your body, especially
those that are particularly tense.**
Do this for a few minutes, until you feel that the physical

tension is released from your body. But do not overdo it, especially if you have any specific physical condition which precludes you from heavy physical activities.

Check whether any part of you still feels particularly tense. If it does, repeat the whole procedure once again. If not, proceed with what you were going to do – do an AT exercise, go to bed, continue with your daily chores, or whatever.

The noise-loosening exercise

This is a useful little exercise for releasing tension from around the vocal cords as well as the throat, particularly for those people who do a lot of talking or public speaking or who feel choked up in their throats and at the top of the chest, or who get the feeling of something being stuck in their throats. (In this last instance I must assume that you have not actually got something physically stuck in your throat! If you think there may be something wrong, consult your GP without delay.) The screaming exercise can also be quite helpful for this feeling.

How do I do it?

Just make any weird or baby noises that come up. Really indulge and enjoy yourself. Do the things that you were prevented from doing as a child. Do it for as long as it feels comfortable.

You can, if you want to, combine this with the motor-loosening exercise. But if you do, make sure that you are not seen by anyone, as they might think that you have really flipped your lid! A much milder and gentler version of the noise-loosening exercise is the simple *humming exercise*.

The humming exercise

Sit or stand, and relax. It does not matter whether you close your eyes or leave them open. Then just **hum any tune you like**. Preferably, allow any natural noises that want to come out, to do so. Try to alter the pitch and the tone of your humming, and then put your hands over different parts of your body. You will find that different humming pitches will vibrate and reverberate in different parts. This is also a good way of trying to offload pain from different parts of the body. However, to be able to vibrate at the pitch of each organ, which this calls for, will take a lot of practice and patience. But there is nothing to stop you doing it!

ANXIETY- AND FEAR-OFFLOADING EXERCISE

This is a simple but effective exercise for getting rid of feelings of anxiety, fear and phobia. Before you start doing the exercise, it is worthwhile making a list of all the people, places and situations that are making you anxious, worried or fearful now, or have done in the past. Apart from giving you a pointer to the sort of things that affect you, this will also indicate how you can cut down the sources and causes of your anxiety – at this stage you can at least avoid them, until you have learnt how to deal with them properly

You can, of course, do this anxiety-offloading exercise either when you are feeling anxious or scared, or when, although you are not having any of these particular feelings, you want to offload past worries and anxieties.

How do I do it?

Sit in a non-AT position. Think of one of the people, places or situations on your list, and **verbalise loudly any thoughts or feelings that come up**, such as 'I am scared and worried', 'I am petrified'. Repeat the phrases as fast as you can. You will find that as you go on repeating them they will eventually merge and you will end up mumbling to yourself. At that point, wait and see if any other phrase comes up.

It is extremely important that if you suffer from any particular phobias – for instance, if you are scared of something specific such as spiders, thunder and lightning, catching AIDS or getting cancer, to name but a few – **you must mention the dreaded word/s.** For unless you do, you will not be able to break through the vicious circle of the phobia.

One of the comments that people suffering from anxiety often make is that if they keep on saying that they are scared of something they will get even more scared or anxious about it. This is quite a reasonable assumption to make; after all, one is usually told to try to forget about the source of one's fear or anxiety. However, unfortunately here is where the root of the problem lies! If you try to forget about your fear or its source, all that will happen is that the memory and the fearful feelings associated with it get even more deeply buried in the unconscious, and thus go on causing even more problems, either in the way of feelings of overt anxiety, fear or panic, or, worse still, manifestations of such physical symptoms as palpitations, headaches or tightness in the throat or chest.

But if we manage to verbalise, offload, **externalise** the feelings of anxiety – whether or not we become aware of the thoughts, experiences or memories related to the causes of it – then those feelings leave us and dissipate into the air. **And once they are out of us, they are not stuck in the unconscious knocking to get out; they are out and away, and consequently will not cause any short- or long-term problems.** As a result of this offloading process we feel refreshed and more content, since those long-standing feelings of anxiety, which are extremely draining, have been removed. DON'T FORGET, though, that you may have a great many reasons for feeling anxious or scared, and hence many sources of anxiety and fear. So it is well worth checking your list of anxiety-producing situations and updating it frequently, so that you can work through them quickly, adequately and systematically.

SADNESS-OFFLOADING EXERCISES

Tears and crying were designed by nature as a means of getting rid of feelings of sadness, depression and grief. Unfortunately however, in the West especially, our uprbringing and our outdated and outmoded sociological norms have made it unacceptable for these very important emotions to be expressed, especially in public and especially by men! It is not only that the demonstration of such emotions is frowned upon, but also that we are expected not to feel them, to pretend, indeed, that we are not feeling anything and to wear the stiff upper lip at all times, though we may be in intense emotional, psychological or physical distress. This is particularly true of my own profession; for one of the lessons that we are taught in medical school is that as doctors we must not get involved with our patients' emotions or feelings.

I do not think that there is any other job or profession in which one is so constantly faced with disease, distress and pain of so many types, and death. Yet we are not supposed to get involved! I cannot honestly see how any conscientious or caring doctor could avoid taking on at least some of the burdens of his or her patients, which can be extraordinarily heart-rending. But we have been taught to repress our feelings and pretend that they do not exist! And when we do repress these feelings of depression or the desire to cry, all we do is store up enormous troubles for ourselves.

The symptoms associated with repressed crying needs are many and varied: they can present in our daily lives in the form of incessant depression, extreme tiredness or listlessness and difficulty with sleeping, especially early-morning waking, or we may just feel generally awful for no apparent reason. This latter symptom can be especially pronounced first thing in the morning, so that even after a long night's sleep we still feel tired, unrested and lethargic. There may be other symptoms that are less obviously associated with the need to offload tears. These include backache, neckache, and inflammation or pain in various joints, ligaments and muscles. Rheumatoid arthritis is a prime example; it is almost as if we are crying into our joints. The other condition, in women, which may be associated with a crying need is problems with periods, especially heavy blood loss. In time you may find other symptoms which for you indicate a need to offload tears. We are all unique, and the symptoms mentioned here by no means constitute an exhaustive list.

The signs of a need to cry may be more hidden still, and may present as a symptom in only a few, or even just one, of the AT exercises. Frontal headaches or feelings of heaviness in the forehead, twitches and tremblings in the muscles of the face and neck, coughing spells, spontaneous, irrational laughing, and frequent and uncomfortable swallowing – all these may crop up during AT.

As I said earlier in this lesson, feelings are very complex and usually interlinked, and we classify them into different categories merely to make it easier to describe them. DON'T FORGET THAT DEPRESSION MAY BE DUE TO REPRESSED RAGE AND

ANGER RATHER THAN TO SADNESS. It is therefore well worth-while trying this and the next exercise for anger too. You may find that some overlapping happens spontaneously, anyway: you may start with the *crying exercise*, which may then lead to the *anger exercise*, and back again – which is perfectly normal.

The most important thing to do in the first instance is to give yourself permission to feel sad, depressed and miserable. Once you have done that, **then give yourself permission to get rid of those feelings.**

Once you have given yourself permission to feel sad and have decided that you want to do something about it, you can proceed. However, there are FOUR GOLDEN RULES that you must observe before you do the crying exercise:

1 **Never practise the crying exercise less than one hour before doing AT,** although it is perfectly all right to do it immediately after your AT session, especially if you have got in touch with strong feelings during it. However, **you must make absolutely sure that you have cancelled properly, before proceeding any further.**

The reason why you do not do the crying exercise before an AT session is that you may not have fully worked through the emotion, memory or whatever, even though you think you have; which means that when you do your AT you may get in touch with a rush of very uncomfortable feelings that are difficult to deal with during the standard exercise. And, likewise, you must cancel properly before you proceed with the crying exercise if you wish to do it after AT, for if you do not, the feelings that you get in touch with may be over-whelming.

2 **Never practise in an autogenic training position,** just in case you accidentally slip into an AT state without realising it, and get in touch with too much all in one go.

3 **Never practise before going to bed,** as you do not particularly want to take to bed with you uncomfortable feelings, memories or experiences with which you may have got in touch, and thereby cause yourself a disturbed night.

4 **Never practise if you are short of time,** for if you stop suddenly, before you have quite finished with that particular episode, you may feel even worse. This may happen, of

course, even if you thought that you had plenty of time but were suddenly disturbed in mid-spate. ALWAYS the unexpected can happen to disrupt even the best laid plans! This in itself does you no harm except for possibly making you uncomfortable until you get another opportunity to repeat the exercise for a longer, adequate time. That's all you need to do to get rid of the left-over feelings.

There are also some technical points worth remembering:

1   The appearance of tears is **not** necessary for the beneficial effects of this exercise. Usually the exercise produces what we call 'dry crying': that is, although there may not have been any actual tears, except perhaps for one or two, one feels as if one has had a cry. Having said that, it is also worth remembering that occasionally you may get in touch with the actual cause of your tears and may want to go on crying for some time. It is important to allow yourself plenty of time for doing the exercise just in case that happens, so that you will not have to terminate it prematurely, thereby depriving yourself of its full benefits. To get in touch with a root cause and offload a lot of tears is a rare enough gift, so we must make the most of it when the opportunity arises.
2   Apart from using this exercise when you are feeling sad and depressed, you can of course, use it when you are not feeling either, in order to get in touch with and offload the backlog of past tears.
3   You can use sad or moving background music if you wish.
4   WARN YOUR FAMILY about what you are up to, so that they do not get worried if they suddenly hear a wailing sound issuing from your direction!
5   Remember that if you are worried about being overheard you can put the radio or the television or both on, bury your face in a pillow, or do the exercise under a duvet if necessary. You can also do it in the shower. REMEMBER THAT WHERE THERE'S A WILL, THERE'S ALWAYS A WAY!
6   Finally, remember that you may not feel any better, or may even feel worse, if you finish your exercise too early or do not do enough of it. So keep on trying until you get it right.

Having observed all these points, you are now ready to proceed. But don't let the 'rat' (§4) tell you that you have taken so much time reading about it that you do not have time actually to do the crying exercise! I have heard that excuse many times.

This is quite a difficult exercise to get into, especially for men who are set in the traditional macho mould which dictates that to cry or show emotions is not manly. So before launching yourself into the full crying exercise described below, it may be worth trying the following two exercises several times in order to warm up!

FIRST, you can do a short noise-loosening exercise (see page 91). You can combine it with the motor-loosening exercise if you want to.

SECONDLY, you can do the following *moaning exercise*.

The moaning exercise

Sit forward in your chair, with your hands resting on your thighs and your eyes closed.
Gently rock backwards and forwards. Initially, this is a conscious effort, but after a short while it becomes automatic. At that point – **start making humming, moaning or groaning noises, or any other sounds of distress that may automatically or unconsciously come up.** Go on doing this, either until you feel better and emptied of your sad feelings, or until you start crying or going into a spontaneous full-blown crying exercise.

Apart from preparing you for the crying exercise and offloading feelings of depression and sadness, THIS IS ALSO A VERY USEFUL LITTLE EXERCISE FOR GETTING RID OF, OR DEALING WITH, PAIN.

The full crying exercise

Sit on the front of your seat. (I favour using the lavatory for this purpose, but you can also use the shower which blocks out an enormous amount of the noise, of course.)
Pretend that you are on stage and have heard some really sad and devastating news. Sob your heart out, making sure that

you use all the muscles of your face, neck, shoulders, upper arms and chest.
Repeat this sequence a few times.

Some people need to do just a short set of crying exercises lasting a few minutes, frequently, during the week. Others find that they need a longer session lasting upwards of 20 minutes, 1 to 3 times a week. Both are fine. Just find your own level and a way of doing it that feels comfortable for you, remembering, though, to let the exercise work itself through completely if you tap a large source of tears. Consider it a great gift if this happens to you.

The laughing exercise

One point that is worth bearing in mind is that laughter can be a façade for underlying tears. So it is hardly surprising that, once we get through the superficial layer of apparent jollity, we may get in touch with an underlying source of tears. So if you find that you have trouble or resistance in doing any of the crying exercises, and especially if you feel the need for it, do try this exercise. It is easy and can be quite fun!

How do I do it?

Sit or stand.
Laugh as loudly as you can for as long as you can! You may find that this leads you on to a crying session. That's perfectly all right. Don't forget that laughing and crying are very similar in that they both utilise more or less the same set of muscles in the face, neck and throat. One great difference between the two, apart from the sound that comes out, is that our conditioning makes the sound of laughter, especially in public, far more acceptable than the sound of crying!

ANGER- AND AGGRESSION-OFFLOADING EXERCISES

Anger is a very powerful emotion, and repressing it uses an enormous amount of energy. Consequently, if we manage to get rid of our anger, we end up with a great deal more positive energy, which we can utilise for whatever we wish. Like sadness, anger is one of the basic natural emotions that we experience from the time that we are babies. However, social norms and conditioning teach us from very early in our childhood that it is not acceptable to get angry, or, more accurately, to exhibit anger. What do we do when a child gets angry and starts having a tantrum? We immediately tell him or her to shut up!

Conditioning against the demonstration of anger goes on incessantly throughout life, and so by the time we are adult we genuinely believe that to show anger is wrong, and become fearul not only of our own anger but also of that of others. Consequently we keep on holding our anger in, so that the container that our bodies constitute gets fuller and fuller. When we reach the limit of our tolerance we suddenly explode, thereby frightening ourselves and others, and reinforcing the notion that anger is a destructive and unacceptable thing, which, if we let it out, will destroy us, those around us and anything else that we hold dear. However, if we go on repressing it and not showing it in any way, eventually a fuse in our system goes and we end up with a nervous breakdown, a stroke, a heart attack or a stomach ulcer, to name but a few possibilities. In my experience, women often find it particularly difficult to exhibit anger, which is considered a more male type of behaviour. Some people repress their anger to such an extent that they do not even feel anger in a situation which by rights should make them angry. In fact, they often pride themselves on never getting angry! Little do they realise that by not doing so they are leaving themselves open to a variety of stress-related or psychosomatic illnesses, including cancer. Repressed anger can also lead to severe depression (anger directed inwards), general and unspecific feelings of unwellness, severe exhaustion, backache, neckache and joint pains, as well as piles (haemorrhoids). Excessive repressed anger can also be associated with feelings of anxiety or guilt which may be quite overwhelming.

The process of doing AT exercises may itself bring on specific symptoms which indicate that you have a need to offload feelings of repressed anger. These symptoms include increased irritability, either between sessions or during the exercise; pain in the left side of the chest, which is often sharp but short-lasting – this is assuming that the individual has no underlying heart disease that could be causing the pains; abdominal pains; headaches; and increased pain and tension in the neck or back. So if you come across any of these symptoms in yourself, be aware that you probably need to offload some anger. However, if the symptoms become persistent and do not respond to what seem to you to be adequate anger exercise sessions, then **you must consult your doctor**, just in case there is an underlying physical condition that needs treatment by other means.

Just as in the crying exercise, **the first important thing is to give yourself permission to feel anger, so that you can then offload it** via one of the following exercises.(You are bound to find one of them socially acceptable.) Of course, it is much easier to undertake the anger exercises when you are actually feeling angry. Do remember, though, that you can use them when you are not feeling angry, in order to get rid of accumulated repressed anger, rage and aggression.

Before you start, it is a good idea to make a list of all the people, places, situations and so on that have made you angry in the past or make you angry now. The list must include the following:

1   God, Christ or any other religious leader (if you believe in any) who you feel may have been the cause of your problems.
2   Anyone you love, including husband, wife, partner, boyfriend, girlfriend, children, or any other relations or friends.
3   Doctors, nurses, or any other health care professional who you feel may have sold you short.
4   Yourself, as we are the commonest cause of our own problems, but tend to forget it and allocate blame to everyone and everything except ourselves!

As with the crying exercise, ther are FOUR GOLDEN RULES that you must observe before undertaking this exercise:

1   **Never do it in an AT position.**
2   **Never do it before going to bed.**
3   **Never do it less than one hour before doing your AT exercises,** although you can do it immediately afterwards, especially if you get in touch with a lot of feelings during your

exercises – always ensure, of course, that you have **cancelled properly** before starting the anger exercise.

4   **Never do it if there is insufficient time,** for if you terminate the exercise before it has run its natural course you may feel somewhat worse, until you repeat the exercise and allow it to run its full course.

As with the crying exercise, apart from the 'rat' and natural reluctance the main factor that deters people from doing these exercises is the worry that they may be overheard. What on earth will people think? See my advice on page 96 about ways of dealing with this problem.

One of the easiest, quietest, and quickest ways of offloading anger and frustration is *screaming into a cushion* (described on page 89).

Anger-offloading exercise 1

Ensure that you have no sharp rings on your fingers.
You may put a cushion on your lap before you start.
Sit forwards in your chair, with your forearms on your thighs and your palms facing upwards.
Close your eyes.
Gently tap the backs of your forearms and hands against your thighs. Initially, the tapping is quite self-conscious. Once it has become semi-automatic and feels right –
– start making a grunting noise. Allow the grunts to get progressively louder and the tapping firmer, and allow your feelings to take over. Go on doing this as long as it feels comfortable, as long as you want to, or until you feel emptied. The more freedom you give to your feelings and their expression, the more you will get out of this exercise.

This may sound a very simple exercise, but it is a powerful one, and lets you get in touch with enormous amounts of rage and anger, especially if memories or incidents from the past come into your mind. If they do, allow them to work through, enabling yourself at the same time to get rid of the feelings associated with them.Remember that once the feelings are out they are off and away, and cause no more trouble in the future.

Anger-offloading exercise 2

This one is based on one of the martial arts techniques. Follow the movements described below, with the help of Figure 9.

Stand up with your elbows bent, arms raised in front of you up to shoulder level, and gather up your thoughts – think, perhaps, of someone or something on your list.
Bring your arms down briskly, straightening your elbows and grunting as loudly as you can.
At the same time bend one knee and lift the same foot off the floor, as if you were breaking a twig across your knee. You can, of course, imagine that you are breaking your enemy's neck or back across your knee! Usually the more extreme your imagination, the more effective the exercise will be.

Repeat this as many times as you can physically manage, or until you feel that you have got rid of your anger. Of course, you may not be able to do this one if you have any sort of physical disability affecting your limbs, or if you suffer from any condition that precludes you from physical activity. You can always do one of the other exercises, which are just as effective. You just have to find the one that suits you and your personality.

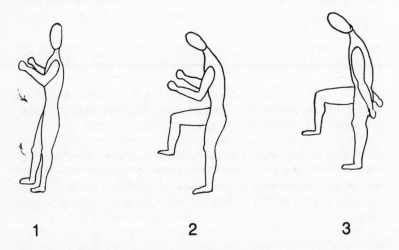

1   2   3

Fig. 9   The positions in anger-offloading exercise 2.

Anger-offloading exercise 3

Sit towards the front of your seat.
Put a soft but firm cushion on your lap.
Think about someone or something on your list.
Concentrate on one and **allow any angry thoughts or words to come up.**
Repeat these thoughts or words as fast as you can, loudly. It is extremely important that you repeat them as loudly as you can, for if you only think them, all that will happen is that they will go straight back into the unconscious and continue in the vicious circle. If you verbalise them loudly, they will be off and away. You can, of course, use any bad language or swearwords that may surface.
Give permission to your feelings to come up.
Once the feelings start surfacing and you get in touch with your real anger, imagine that the person or the situation that angers you is the cushion, and **beat it as hard as you can,** in order to let out the aggression in a physical sense as well. You can also stamp your feet, if you want to.

Go on doing it until you feel emptied of all the anger and aggression – at least for the time being and as far as this particular person or situation is concerned!

Anger-offloading exercise 4

You can do this exercise while walking or stamping about, banging doors, or clattering pots and pans and so on!

Think of your list again. **Pick something or someone out of it, or just use the anger of the moment if something has happened to make you feel angry.**
Conduct a one-sided argument with yourself, imagining your adversary in the room. Say out loud all that you would wish to tell him to his face, using the strongest possible language, including swearwords if you want to. Have a go at him or her and really let off steam. It makes you feel wonderful afterwards!

The intensity of anger felt can be expressed more or less mildly in statements such as 'I don't like you' or 'I hate you', or it can be experienced as a desire to perform such violent actions as torturing or even killing the other person. Don't think that you are mad or abnormal if you have such vicious feelings towards your adversary. Most of us get these feelings from time to time, but because nobody admits to them, or freely discusses them, we think that we are the only ones and that we must be very wicked to think of such things. After all, our upbringing tells us that ideally we should behave like saints all the time! Unfortunately, life is far from ideal for most of us; but it is usually the case that if we express verbally and loudly, and safely, through any of these exercises, the violent thoughts that we may be having, the less likely we are to act them out in reality.

Another common fear when doing any of these exercises is that we will go mad, or go over the top, and not be able to control our actions. Remember that there is no way that you will be able to go beyond the limit that your mind wants to take you to, and feels safe with. We have an enormous number of self-preservation mechanisms and defences in our minds which will stop us going to a point that we feel uncertain about or unsafe with.

Some people worry that if they do all this they will not be able to face in real life the person who is the focus of their anger. In fact this could not be further from the truth. This question often crops up. In fact, the very same worry was expressed to me by one of my staff when she was doing AT. She was having a great deal of trouble with her teenage daughter at the time, and she felt that if she went through this exercise and said what she really thought of her daughter, she would never let her back into the house again! However, after my reassurance, she tried the exercise on a number of occasions. Contrary to her expectations, she found that her feelings towards her daughter changed positively, and for the first time in a long while they started talking to each other and beginning to understand each other. Their relationship now is the closest and the most loving that it has ever been.

I could cite numerous examples like this, which is hardly surprising. When we carry a lot of anger, it chokes us and blocks the channels of communication. We are afraid that if we start discussing something, particularly some contentious issue, we will come rapidly to the boil; and that the container that is already full of all our repressed emotions will overflow, that we will explode and say hurtful things that we do not really mean, and so spoil or destroy everything that is good around us or in our relationship. However, the contrary is usually true. If we offload small amounts of the anger that we have accumulated over the years, and gradually begin to empty the container, then it will take a lot more to get us to boiling point; and for this reason we will not reach that point, unless the provocation is extraordinarily great. When we gain the confidence that we are not going to explode and spoil everything, we find it a lot easier to communicate with the people around us. And as we relax, so will they, for the whole thing has a ripple effect: our relaxation and lack of anger will affect those around us and thus open further the lines of communication.

I am sure that you will find lots of reasons and occasions for letting off steam, using any one of the above exercises, and that you will feel the benefits of it. Although you may feel exhausted immediately after a good anger exercise, you usually feel great after a few minutes' rest. You will find that you feel highly energised, and that all the heavy, lethargic or exhausted feelings that you may have been experiencing beforehand will have disappeared. THIS IS HOW YOU CONVERT THE NEGATIVE ENERGY OF THIS VERY POWERFUL EMOTION INTO A POSITIVE AND ENERGISING ONE.

SUMMARY

Anger-offloading exercise 1
Sit forwards in your chair with your forearms on your thighs. Close your eyes.
With your palms upturned, gently tap your forearms and hands against your thighs.
Grunt at the same time.
Make the tapping firmer and the grunts louder as you get into the exercise. Let your feelings come out.
Go on doing this until you feel emptied of feelings, or until you feel tired.

Anger-offloading exercise 2
Stand up with your elbows bent.

Think of your list, perhaps, and pick someone or something from it.

Briskly straighten your elbows and bend one knee, bringing the same foot off the floor as if to break a twig across your knee.

Grunt loudly at the same time.

Repeat this until you are tired or until you feel that you have exhausted your anger.

Anger-offloading exercise 3

Sit forwards in your chair, with a cushion on your lap.

Think of someone on your list and put him into the cushion.

Say out loud all the angry thoughts or words that may come up. Really let your feelings out.

Beat the cushion with your hands and fists. And stamp your feet, if you like.

Anger-offloading exercise 4

Sit, stand or stamp about.

Think of someone or something on your list, or just use the anger of the moment.

Have a passionate one-sided argument, imagining that your adversary is actually in the room and can hear you! Let him really have it, using any language, including swearwords, that may come up. Usually the stronger the emotions and the language, the more quickly the source of your anger is disposed of.

The retching exercise

Like many old sayings, 'You make me sick to the pit of my stomach' or 'I am sick at the sight of you' have particular significance as far as repressed emotions are concerned. There are times when we do indeed feel sick at certain incidents, memories and so on, and psychological factors play an important role in generating those feelings of nausea. For instance, when we unexpectedly come across an accident or are suddenly shocked by something, we may feel sick, although there is no physical reason why we should.

You may experience feelings of nausea or actually feel the need to vomit during your AT, if you get in touch with very deep emotions that you have repressed into the pit of your stomach (at the level of the solar plexus, explained on page 119). If that happens, you can get tremendous relief by performing this exercise. (We must assume, here, that you are not suffering from any physical illness or are on any drugs that could make you feel sick.)

There are FOUR GOLDEN RULES that you must observe:

1 **Never do this exercise if you are suffering from any sort of stomach trouble, such as an ulcer or a hiatus hernia.**
2 **Never do this exercise within two hours of eating,** as the object of the exercise is not to make you sick but to offload the tension and tightness that you have repressed into the muscles of your gullet and stomach.
3 **Always consult a doctor,** even if you have no stomach or bowel trouble that you know of, **if you find that the symptoms of nausea and actual vomiting do not resolve quickly with this exercise.**
4 **Only** do this exercise if you **need** to offload feelings of nausea. Don't do it routinely, as it can cause pain and inflammation of the gullet.

How do I do it?

Sit or stand in front of the lavatory or wash-basin.
Take your glasses off if you wear any.
Put one finger at the back of your throat, and feel yourself retch.
Do this several times, until you feel that the nausea has gone.

You may find that while you are doing this you remember the event that was the cause of your feelings. At the end of a good session you usually find that your eyes water and your nose runs, but you feel good in yourself! It may not appear at first glance that you could possibly feel good after such an exercise. This has only to do with the social conditioning that tells us that retching or vomiting is an awful event. The more revulsion you feel about it initially, usually the more you need to do it.

This is also quite a useful exercise for those who have undergone attempted strangulation, rape or suffocation, as it can help to offload the tight feelings that they may be feeling in their throats, for instance.

THE FORGIVENESS AND COMFORTING EXERCISE

It is often very difficult to forgive either ourselves or others who we may feel have done us wrong. Our anger and inability to forgive someone who has committed an act of violence against us, whether physical, emotional or psychological, may be perfectly justifiable. However, it is important to bear in mind that we can only become truly at peace with ourselves when we have managed to extricate from our minds the painful thorns of negative emotions or memories. It is often by doing so that we can make enough space in our hearts and lives to allow in new, fresh and joyful experiences, as well as unconditional love and light. We will know instinctively when that happens, as our whole attitude towards ourselves and all those around us will change, and will be tinged with the light and delicate touch of joy and beauty, rather than with the dark and ugly shadow of bitterness and recrimination.

It can take an enormously long time and a great deal of perseverance, patience and love before we achieve a state that permits us to genuinely forgive our adversary, whether the offence be perceived or real. At first we may need that hatred or anger to help us to cope with the situation that generated it in the first place. However, once we start working on ourselves and on our deeper being, we usually find that we get into a state of mind that favours forgiveness, as we realise that it is only by forgiving that we can let go and free ourselves of all the negative, unrewarding energies of the past that hold us back and so slow us down on our journey towards transformation and eventual freedom. Furthermore, when we reach that state we may also wish to comfort, support and congratulate ourselves on having achieved such a breakthrough in our journey towards self-awareness, growth and emancipation. Do remember, though, that sometimes the person that you get in touch with is the child within you, who needs all the comfort, support and nurturing that he or she may never have had in the past, and the absence of which may be a major contributory factor towards your present problems.

You may enter the state of forgiveness either when you have successfully completed one of the exercises already mentioned, or at any time in your life when, as a result of a great deal of inner work, you realise that you no longer need to hold on to the negative and painful experiences or emotions of the past. When that happens, then you will be able to proceed with the following *forgiveness and comforting exercise.*

How do I do it?

Get hold of your favourite teddy-bear or doll if you have one, or a cushion or pillow. REMEMBER THAT THE TEDDY-BEAR OR DOLL MAY HAVE BEEN YOUR SOLE WITNESS AND COMFORTER AT YOUR MOMENTS OF GREATEST NEED AND VULNERABILITY, WHEN YOU EXPERIENCED YOUR MOST DISTRESSING THOUGHTS AND NIGHTMARES, HORRIFIC MEMORIES, PAINS OR SILENT SCREAMS. Having done that, then **sit or lie down** – whichever feels more comfortable.
Hold your favourite object in your arms and rock very gently backwards and forwards.
Say all the forgiving, calming or comforting thoughts or words that spontaneously come up.
Go on in this way **until you feel that you have emptied yourself of all that needs to be said or done, and that this chapter in your life's experience is closed.**

Then rest for a few minutes, until you have gathered your thoughts and can return to the present. Allow yourself to fall asleep, if that is what you feel like. Don't forget that you have worked immensely hard to get into the state of mind that permitted you to do what you have just done. Enjoy for as long as possible the peace and tranquillity that will probably descend upon you at this time.

You can repeat this exercise as often as you feel the need or the desire to do so. But remember that **there is no point in doing it unless you are genuinely ready to move on and change**, as you will gain nothing from it if you are not yet ready to go through with the forgiveness process.

OTHER WAYS OF OFFLOADING

Some of you may have difficulty with one or more of the exercises just described. **The crucial thing is that you give yourself permission to feel**, and that you realise that there is nothing wrong with that, irrespective of whether the feelings are of depression, sadness, anger, rage or frustration, or of love and happiness. The other extremely important point is that once you have started taking note of your feelings **you must find ways of expressing them that feel comfortable and acceptable to you**. If you find that a particular exercise mentioned earlier in the lesson is effective for you, all well and good. If not, there are other things that you can do in order to offload or deal with your emotions and feelings. For instance, you can seek the help of some other kind of therapist, such as a *counsellor*, a *co-counsellor* or a *psychotherapist* (individual or group). There are a great many kinds of therapy, and you must find the type that suits you and your personality. (See Appendix 1, 2 and Further Reading for further information and useful books.) Here are some more offloading activities that you may like to try:

Deep externalisation work   Some people may find that in order to deal with their emotions and feelings at a much deeper level they need to work with a trained therapist in a safe and loving atmosphere, where they can act out feelings of severe anger or rage, for instance, by beating or tearing up telephone directories. **This must not be done without supervision**. The Shanti Nilaya organisation in the United States, founded on the work of Dr Elisabeth Kübler-Ross in this field, runs Life, Death and Transition residential workshops at locations around Britain, where therapists help participants to get in touch with deep, repressed, and often painful emotions and work through them. Details of the work of the organisation, which is represented by Shanti Nilaya in Britain, will be found in Appendix 1.

Painting is important, particularly if you hit a block. So get painting! You do not have to know anything about it – in fact, the less you know and the less you think you can do, the more you will get out of this form of therapy and offloading. It certainly does not mean sitting down and drawing or painting a pretty picture. The best way of offloading through the medium of art is to use water-soluble paints or ordinary lead pencil and paint or draw as fast as you can whatever comes into your mind or through your brush onto the paper. If you like this way of expressing moods and feelings, you can, of course, see a qualified art therapist. And there are books that will give you an idea of what the various shapes that you produce may symbolise.

There is, in fact, a kind of art therapy that is sometimes utilised in conjunction with autogenic training. It is called the creative mobilisation technique (CMT, for short). Unfortunately, there are no experienced trainers in Britain at the time of going to press, so I am not going to discuss it in detail. Suffice it to say that the trainees use several basic colours, a 1½-in. paintbrush and large sheets of newspaper! You aim to fill a whole sheet, using at least five different colours in two minutes. You do fifteen paintings in half an hour. The course is normally run over an eight-week period, the trainee doing at least three half-hour sessions at home during the week, between his sessions with the therapist. The paintings are then interpreted jointly by the trainee and therapist. The premise is that, as one is doing the whole thing so fast, one draws one's imagery and colours from the unconscious, and the interpretation of these over a period of time gives an indication of possible blocks and helps one to work through them.

Music is another great activity for the expression of emotions. You can use any instrument for the purpose, and you can undertake music therapy if that appeals to you.

Dancing is an excellent way of offloading tensions, especially physical ones. There are special meditative and sacred dances that constitute, for some people, extremely powerful ways of offloading tension and developing relaxation.

Writing has already been mentioned as a means of expressing one's emotions. Although writing essays, letters and dramas can be helpful, the most effective way of utilising writing for this purpose is to write whatever comes into your mind as fast as you can and not to worry about grammatical accuracy and so on. The rapid associations of thoughts, memories and images with the feelings related to them that come to the surface are of the utmost importance. It is these associations and the related feelings that help you to deal with whatever the problem may be.

Drama Techniques using puppets and psychodrama, amongst other things, can also help you to get in touch with and offload unworked-through negative feelings, emotions and memories.

Fun, creativity and transformation workshops As mentioned earlier in this lesson, both the release of the so-called 'negative' emotions and the utilisation of positive emotions lead to improvement in the health and the healing powers of the individual. The author and his associate have devised workshops (weekend or five-day residential), in which a warm, safe, comfortable and at times party atmosphere is created. In this friendly environment the participants are encouraged to use a variety of techniques – including games, pictures, puppets, drawing, clay, masks, music, dance (creative as well as meditative), relaxation, visualisation and guided imagery – in order to work through some of their negative emotions and, by using positive emotions and creativity, enhance their progress towards better health. No expertise is required: the only criterion is willingness to 'have a go'. The workshops thus promote fun and enjoyment while doing deep emotional work designed to lead to transformation and a better quality of life. Transformation in this context means changing old and familiar patterns of behaviour to more positive and constructive ones. Unless we do this, we cannot progress to healing and true healthy living. For details see Appendix 1, p. 293.

These are just a few suggestions. You may already have your own ways of dealing with and expressing emotions. That's fine, as long as you use them to their best advantage.

Lesson 6 Continue with the breathing exercise

I hope that you have had no major problems with the introduction of the heartbeat exercise, or if you have, that you
have managed to deal with them via at least one of the ways
described in lesson 5. If you still find that the incorporation of
'My heartbeat is calm and regular' causes you discomfort or
anxiety, there are two main ways of proceeding.

If the symptoms are not too acute, proceed with the
exercise but reduce the number of repetitions. However, if
you find that they are still pretty uncomfortable, either go on
working slowly and gently with that phrase for a while longer
or, preferably, leave it out for a while, carry on with the
breathing exercise, and see how you get on. If you find that this
exercise is relaxing and comfortable, just introduce the heartbeat exercise from time to time, for perhaps one repetition in
one exercise, and see what happens. If the symptoms recur, it
means that you still have not worked through the associated
unresolved feelings. Leave it out for a while longer, then keep
on introducing it from time to time. However, note that for a
variety of reasons **some people have to leave out one or more of
the phrases or formulae altogether. This does not matter, and
does not reduce the ultimate effectiveness of the standard (full)
AT exercises. If you do not leave the offending phrase out,
though, and try to push your way through it, then your AT will
certainly suffer and you will not get the full benefits.** You have
to be kind, gentle and sensible with yourself, as I keep
repeating! Everything has to work through at its own pace for
it to be effective, and YOU CANNOT HURRY THINGS ALONG. The
ONLY way that you can help to speed things up is by dealing
with and working through the repressed or unresolved problems, either by using one or more of the offloading exercises
(lesson 5) or by seeking the help of a professional counsellor
or therapist.

Although most people find the *Breathing exercise* particularly relaxing and helpful, some trainees may occasionally have difficulties with it. This can include those who have a respiratory disease such as chronic bronchitis, emphysema and asthma, and those who have had some form of 'near-death experience', particularly through the interference of the breathing mechanism, such as near-drowning, choking, strangulation or suffocation.

Therefore, if this includes you, it is **essential that you start this exercise with extreme caution**. This means that you introduce it just once into one exercise, and see what happens. If you have no problems, then gradually increase the number of repetitions. If you find that you do have problems, which may range from very mild to severe, follow the instruction already given: reduce the sensations either by reducing the number of repetitions or by leaving the phrase out altogether for a while; then reintroduce it slowly, and perhaps intermittently.

A number of relaxation and meditation techniques utilise breathing as a part of the relaxation process, and try to alter it to suit their specific purposes. The way we utilise it in AT, however, is totally different. **In this exercise we do not try to do anything at all with our breathing**, and hence the rather nonsensical-sounding phrase that we use: **'It breathes me'**. As usual, we incorporate it between the 'heartbeat exercise' and 'My neck and shoulders are heavy'. Since we are not trying to do anything with our breathing, instead of concentrating on our chests while quietly repeating the phrase to ourselves **we concentrate on the breath that comes in and out of our noses or mouths**, depending on whether we normally nose- or mouth-breathe. At the same time we remain passive observers, and watch what happens to the rest of our bodies and minds.

At this stage, provided that you are not having any difficulties, you can go on doing your exercises **without cancelling** between sets. By doing this you will find that you start going a lot deeper, particularly during the second or third set. You can also gradually increase the length of the exercises from the 10 minutes or so each session that you have been spending so far to an eventual 20 minutes, or longer if you wish. You will now be able to utilise the technique fully on the bus, in waiting rooms, or wherever.

The other thing that you can do at this stage is stay in any part of the exercise for a few minutes and really enjoy it, especially if you get into a deep and pleasant state – which is bound to happen more frequently, the more you practise your exercises. If you do decide to stay in a part of the exercise that feels good to you, you can prolong your stay in two ways:

1   By saying the same phrase repeatedly. For instance, you go into a deep state during the second set of the 'heartbeat exercise'. Keep repeating 'My heartbeat is calm and regular' until you want to continue, then proceed with the rest of the phrases, and cancel after 'I am at peace'.
2   If you are in a state of mental silence – which can happen if you are very deeply relaxed – you remain in that state until your concentration starts wandering. Then move on to the rest of the exercise, and cancel as usual.

Remember at this stage that you DO NOT have to slavishly and regimentally count the number of repetitions as you go along, as long as you say each phrase several times – anything from 2 to 5 is all right. It is important to allow the whole relaxation process to float along, so that you get the most out of it. You may also find that you repeat one phrase more or less than another: for instance, you may say, 'My arms and legs are heavy and warm' three times, 'My heartbeat is calm and regular' four times, and 'It breathes me' twice. This kind of irregularity at this stage is perfectly acceptable, since by allowing your mind to freewheel you are more likely to get into a truly passive state, rather than regimentally counting 'One, two, three', which will keep you in the actively concentrating, conscious state.

The other important thing to remember is that from now on, as you become progressively more able to relax, you may get in touch with colours or lights in your deep state: that is, you may become aware of them in your mind's eye. The colours may take the form, for instance, of a combination of coloured squares, or starburst effects such as fireworks produce. If you allow this state to develop and go passively with it, you may find that eventually the whole of your field of vision is filled with the same colour or coloured light. This is just an example of what might happen – the process might be totally different for you. IT IS PERFECTLY ALL RIGHT TO

CONTINUE WITH YOUR AT WITHOUT CANCELLING IF YOU START GETTING IN TOUCH WITH COLOURS OR LIGHTS, IRRESPECTIVE OF THE FORMS THEY MAY TAKE, AS ALL IT MEANS IS THAT YOU HAVE GONE VERY DEEPLY INTO YOUR AT STATE.

So the exercise for the next week is as follows:

Get into a correct AT position.
Scan.
Take your attention to your dominant arm (right or left), become a passive observer of your body and mind, and see what happens as you go through the following formulae:
'My right (left) arm is heavy' – **once.**
'My arms and legs are heavy and warm' – **3 times** (approximately, from now on).
'My heartbeat is calm and regular' – **3 times.**
'It breathes me' – **3 times.**
'My neck and shoulders are heavy' – **3 times.**
'I am at peace' – **3 times.**
Repeat the whole of this exercise 2 or 3 times (with the exception of the scan), staying in and luxuriating in any part where you feel particularly relaxed and comfortable.
Cancel.

Remember that the deeper you go, the more likely it is that you will become totally unaware of your body. You may also very occasionally feel as if you are actually standing above your body. This is what we call an *out-of-the-body experience*, and it is usually extremely pleasant as long as you are aware of it and do not get scared or panicky about it. It is a perfectly safe state, and you will return to total normality as soon as you cancel, although you may have to cancel two or three times, because of the very deep level of the experience. The other feeling that you may get if you go very deeply into an AT state is one of total weightlessness, which may make you feel that you are going to lift off the surface on which you are practising your AT. This is sometimes referred to as *levitation*; and it is another perfectly harmless, and often very pleasant, state to be in. You will return to normal consciousness and sensations as soon as you have cancelled, firmly and briskly – you may have to cancel more than once. These sensations are uncommon, and only happen when we are totally relaxed at all levels. But it is worth knowing about them, so that if they do happen you do not worry.

SUMMARY OF LESSON 6

Get into an AT position.
Scan.
Take your mind to your dominant arm, and repeat:
'My right (left) arm is heavy' – once.
'My arms and legs are heavy and warm' – 3 times.
'My heartbeat is calm and regular' – 3 times.
'It breathes me' – 3 times.
'My neck and shoulders are heavy' – 3 times.
'I am at peace' – 3 times.
Repeat the whole exercise 2 or 3 times (excluding the scan).
Cancel.

Homework
Do the above exercise 3 times a day using the different AT positions.
Try some of the offloading exercises (lesson 5).
Keep repeating 'My neck and shoulders are heavy' frequently during the day, as a partial exercise to top up your relaxation and to break the cycle of stress in between the exercises.
Remember to do the short exercise (lesson 1) if you are short of time or in touch with a lot of powerful emotions or pain.
Remember: **Do not cancel at night, before going to sleep.**

Lesson 7   Add the abdominal warmth exercise

How did you get on with the last exercise? I hope you had no problems with it. But if you did get in touch with some anxiety, for instance, which may have made the exercise uncomfortable, you should apply the principles discussed at the beginning of the last lesson, as they apply equally to this one.

For this session we concentrate on the abdomen (stomach), and the *solar plexus*. Perhaps you have heard of this region of the body, but don't know where it is! If you were a boxer you would certainly know about it, for if you were hit hard there you would be knocked unconscious, as the solar plexus is the headquarters of the autonomic nervous system (page 5), and a sudden blow to that area would momentarily paralyse the functioning of the heart and other vital organs.

Before going any further it is important to observe some precautions, especially if you have any problems with your stomach. Although this exercise is usually quite useful in helping to deal with and heal stomach ulcers and any other problems in that region, you must appreciate that occasionally any symptoms of pain, discomfort or indigestion that you may have can get worse. So if you have any symptoms, **it is extremely important that you discontinue this exercise if your symptoms get worse or if you develop other unpleasant feelings or side-effects**. If the symptoms are not too uncomfortable you can always reduce the strength of the exercise, either by reducing the number of repetitions or by introducing the word 'slightly' before 'warm', as discussed in previous lessons (see page 76, for example).

I will first describe the solar plexus and its functions, and then with the help of Figure 10 I will explain exactly where it is, so that **in time** you will be able to get in touch with it. Remember,

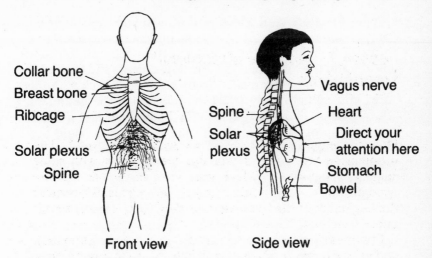

Fig. 10   The position of the solar plexus.

though, that this information has been greatly simplified in order to make it generally comprehensible.

The solar plexus is situated more or less at the top of the abdomen and the lower part of the chest. It is the striped and patterned area in Figure 10. As you can see, it covers quite a large area. It intricately surrounds a great many structures, including the main blood-carrying artery in the body, called the aorta, and the oesophagus (gullet). From the solar plexus radiate out numerous nerves to all the vital organs in the body – which are controlled by the autonomic nervous system (see page 5) – such as the heart, lungs, stomach and bowels, as well as other parts such as arteries and veins, bones, joints and muscles. This, the 'headquarters' of the autonomic nervous system, is a very important area. It is a complex junction box, where all the information to and from the organs and tissues is interchanged and relayed to the brain through a number of interconnecting pathways such the vagus nerve. As you are probably aware, the brain controls, directly through the nervous pathways and indirectly through various chemicals and hormones in the blood, all the functions of every organ and tissue in the body, including the immune system, the proper functioning of which is of utmost importance for the proper defence of the body against infections and cancerous growth. It is through the interconnection between the solar plexus and the brain that the fine adjustments and control of all the vital organs is made. So by getting in touch with this area you can indirectly affect the function of the brain and, through that, everything else in the body. The close involvement of autogenic training with the solar plexus could partially explain why it has such a powerful effect on all the systems of the body, promoting self-regulation and self-healing in those who undertake it.

How do I locate my solar plexus?

In order to locate the solar plexus, we aim for roughly the centre of it. (But don't forget that you have already been accessing it indirectly by getting in touch with your heart and breathing.) Put a finger on the soft part at the top of the abdomen, at the junction of the two halves of the rib-cage (see Figure 10). Then draw a straight line in your mind's eye between that point and an equivalent point on your back. The mid-point of that line is roughly where the solar plexus is situated. In an average slim person it is about 4 in. from both front and back. Don't forget that it occupies a large expanse, and as long as you take your mind roughly to that area you are bound to get in touch with it in time. It is not an easy area to get in touch with, though, despite its importance, and most people have difficulty with it initially. It may be quite some time before you manage it. BE PATIENT WITH YOURSELF.

The phrase that we use for this exercise is '**My solar plexus is warm**', and while we repeat it quietly to ourselves we take our attention to the region of the solar plexus and watch what happens to the whole of the body. We introduce it after the breathing exercise and before the phrase 'My neck and shoulders are heavy'. Don't forget that if you get very strong reactions or if you suffer from a stomach disorder such as an ulcer, you can reduce the strength of the formula either by reducing the number of repetitions or by saying 'My solar plexus is *slightly* warm'. Do remember, too, that although you say, 'My solar plexus is warm', you must sit back and watch what sensations you *actually* feel in that area, as they will depend to a large extent on what quantity of repressed emotions, memories and so on you have stored there. As you will be aware by now, we have been going progressively deeper into ourselves, and this is the deepest level at which you can store anything.

You may find that at first the area feels cold or black. It may feel as if there is a hollow, a hole or a block of ice there. It may feel like a tight knot, especially if you carry a lot of your repressed tensions or emotions at that level. Just observe what your feelings and emotions are. Eventually it will all work through, and you will start feeling warm there. However, it can take a long time. It took someone I know seven months to work through all her emotional, marital and other problems, before she started having any feelings of warmth at this level.

Apart from uncomfortable feelings, you may also start having vivid dreams and nightmares as the unconscious begins to offload and de-stress itself. So if the feelings are too intense or uncomfortable, start gently by saying the new phrase perhaps just once in one exercise, and gradually increase the number of repetitions as the whole thing becomes more comfortable. As with all the other formulae, you may even have to leave the phrase out for a short while, or altogether, if you find it particularly uncomfortable. Don't worry if you have to leave this one out. The final outcome, as far as the benefits of AT are concerned, will be the same as it would have been if you had included it, although it may take somewhat longer. Of course, another way of dealing with these feelings is to use the offloading exercises freely (lesson 5). You are particularly likely to have to use the retching exercise at this point. But do observe the precautions associated with it.

Having taken into account all the above comments, and provided that you are not having any major problems, the full exercise for the next week is as follows:

Get into a correct AT position.
Scan.
Take your attention to your dominant arm (right or left), just

become a passive observer of your whole being, and see what happens as you go through the following formulae:
'My right (left) arm is heavy' – **once.**
'My arms and legs are heavy and warm' – **3 times.**
'My heartbeat is calm and regular' – **3 times.**
'It breathes me' – **3 times.**
'My solar plexus is warm' – **3 times.**
'My neck and shoulders are heavy' – **3 times.**
'I am at peace' – **3 times.**
Repeat the whole exercise (excluding the scan) **at least 3 times. Cancel.**

Keep good but brief notes of your experiences.

Remember that you do not necessarily have to slavishly repeat each phrase 3 times at this stage, and that it is best to float with the phrases and repeat each one as many times as seems appropriate. You may also find that by this stage you are drifting from one phrase into another, prompted by the sensations in the different parts of your body. For instance, you repeat 'My arms and legs are heavy and warm' until you become aware of your heartbeat; then you drift into that and repeat 'My heartbeat is calm and regular', until you become aware of your breathing, and so on.

Homework
Repeat the above exercises at least 3 times during the day, using all 3 main AT positions.
Use the neck and shoulders exercise repeatedly during the day, to top up your relaxation and to break off the daily cycle of accumulating stress.
Use the offloading exercises freely.
Use the short exercise (lesson 1) as often as you can, especially if you are short of time.

Lesson 8 Add the forehead-cooling exercise

How have you been getting on with the solar plexus exercise? If you have not had any major problems – which could even include your not having been able to locate it yet or feel any warmth in it – then you can proceed with this next exercise. Or perhaps you would like to carry on trying the solar plexus one until you are quite definitely in touch with it. Whatever you decide to do is perfectly all right. After all, you are in the process of trying to empower yourself, to become responsible for yourself and to exercise your options. If you have been getting in touch with a lot of uncomfortable feelings, emotions, memories or anxieties, you can deal with them as described in lesson 5.

One of the main reasons for choosing the formula 'My forehead is cool' and its variants to complete the series of exercises, was the fact that in the early days, when no effective tranquillisers were available, the application of cool compresses to the forehead of the agitated patients was found to have a marked relaxing effect, especially if he or she was immersed in a bath of warm water. I hope that by the time you get to this point, after all the previous exercises, you will have a warm body, and that the introduction of this exercise will enhance your state of relaxation.

The forehead is NOT just the bit above the eyes. When we think of it in this context, our minds should run from one temple just above the ears, right across the forehead, to the other temple above the other ear. The phrase that we use is '**My forehead is cool**'. You can also use the phrase, '**My forehead is cool and clear**' or '**My forehead is cool and light**'. I personally prefer the second; I find it functional as well as pleasing because it helps me to clear some of the clutter that seems to fill my head from time to time! But the choice is yours. The important thing is that **you do not want to make it cold**, for if you do that you may end up with a headache. If you get any sensations at all, it should be like a gentle breeze on a warm sunny day. You can get a feel of it by gently blowing on the back of your hand. Go on – try it!

Despite getting this gentle feeling, or no sensations at all, you may still find that you end up with a frontal headache. This does not mean that the exercise is not right for you. On the contrary, it may mean that you are getting in touch with some emotions, especially sadness, and you need to offload that through one of the exercises in lesson 5. You may also become aware of discomfort if you suffer from chronic sinusitis or catarrh. If the symptoms are too uncomfortable, either leave out this formula for a bit while working on the offloading exercises, or if they are not too bad, reduce the strength either by reducing the number of repetitions or by saying '*slightly* cool'.

So your exercise for the next week will be:

Get into the correct AT position. (Have you checked your position recently, to ensure that you are doing it properly?)
Scan.
Take your attention to your dominant arm (right or left), become a passive observer of yourself, and see what happens as you go through the exercise.
'My right (left) arm is heavy' – **once.**
'My arms and legs are heavy and warm' – **3 times.**
'My heartbeat is calm and regular' – **3 times.**
'It breathes me' – **3 times.**
'My solar plexus is warm' – **3 times.**
'My forehead is cool and clear (light)' – **3 times.**
'My neck and shoulders are heavy' – **3 times.**
'I am at peace' – **3 times.**
Repeat the above (with the exception of the scan) **as many times as you wish.**
Cancel.

Remember to give yourself the time and the space that you so richly deserve, to love yourself and to enjoy what you are doing.

Homework
Repeat the above exercise at least 3 times a day, using different positions.

Use the offloading exercises as and when you require them.
Use the neck and shoulders exercise repeatedly during the day, not only to top up your relaxation but also to break the cycle of stress and prevent it from building up.
Use the short exercise (lesson 1) if you haven't enough time to do a full AT exercise, or if you are particularly angry, distressed or in pain.

Lesson 9   Positive affirmations

You have now had the full series of exercises, and I hope that by now you are able to get into a deeply relaxed state within yourself. If you find that you are still unable to relax thoroughly, or that your concentration wanders, don't worry about it. All this will come with time, practice and patience. All of us tend to be too impatient with ourselves, to expect far too much and to get irritated if we do not achieve immediately everything that we set out to do. The bad habits of years take a while to change, modify or overcome So be patient, gentle and loving with yourself.

You have reached a very exciting part of your exercises. Once you get into that deep, healing space within yourself, you can utilise it to reaffirm the positive things that you like about yourself, or to deal with or get rid of the negative things about yourself that you wish to change or modify; and, finally, you can use that space to try to develop or achieve new aims and to help yourself to improve and grow. This is where *positive affirmations* come in. They are short, pithy sentences that encapsulate your particular need of the moment, or a long-standing problem, and that you will learn to incorporate into your exercises. I will give examples of the sort of sentences and phrases that you can use, especially in Part 3, but it is important that you learn how to make up your own.

How do I make up my own positive affirmations?

There are FIVE SIMPLE RULES that you must observe in making up your own:

1   **Make the sentences simple.**
2   **Make them short and concise.**
3   **Make them positive in concept.** This does not mean that you must never use the words 'no' or 'not', as sometimes you can make your phrases even more positive by doing so.

4 **Make the phrases definitive, and use the present tense**: for example, 'I know I am confident', and NOT 'I will be confident', or 'I will lose weight after my holidays!', which is a phrase that one of my trainees used – without any benefits, needless to say!

5 Introducing the phrase, '**I know**', before your main phrase or sentence, often makes it feel even more positive. (Some people do not like to use it, though, and it is not essential.) You will have to find out by trial and error what suits you and your personality. Certainly, you may find that if a goal is too difficult to achieve all in one go, you have to approach it in stages.

Where do I incorporate the positive affirmations in my exercises?

Let's assume that you lack confidence, and wish to use the phrase, 'I know I am confident'. There are two main ways of incorporating it:

1 **If you want to achieve something quickly** – for example, you have an interview in a couple of weeks and want to boost your confidence – **introduce the phrase between each of the standard AT phrases, repeating it several times.** So after getting into position and scanning, the formula will be:

'My right (left) arm is heavy' – **once.**
'I know I am confident' – **several times.**
'My arms and legs are heavy and warm' – **3 times.**
'I know I am confident' – **several times.**
'My heartbeat is calm and regular' – **3 times.**
'I know I am confident' – **several times.**
And so on until the end of the set of exercises as far as 'I am at peace', and then **cancel.**

2 This way of incorporating your special phrase is usually more appropriate for **longer-term benefit. Incorporate the phrase between** 'My forehead is cool and clear' **and** 'My neck and shoulders are heavy'. So getting into position and scanning, the exercise will go:

'My right (left) arm is heavy' – **once.**
'My arms and legs are heavy and warm' – **3 times.**

'My heartbeat is calm and regular' – **3 times.**
'It breathes me' – **3 times.**
'My solar plexus is warm' – **3 times.**
'My forehead is cool and clear' – **3 times.**
'I know I am confident' – **several times.**
'My neck and shoulders are heavy' – **3 times.**
'I am at peace' – **3 times.**
Repeat it all 2–4 times.
Cancel.

It is best to start off with just one positive affirmation, giving it a week or two to see what it feels like. If you are using the second method described in this lesson, you cannot expect these phrases to work very quickly initially. They usually take about four weeks before you notice the difference, depending to some extent on what you are trying to achieve. However, there are TWO EXCEPTIONS to this. One is when you use the first method described, and the other is when you use a formula to increase your energy level. A phrase like 'I am full of energy and vitality' seems to work very quickly and you must **never use it at night**, unless you intend to have an active and sleepless night.

Once you have mastered the technique of introducing your own phrases, you can use up to a maximum of three together in one exercise, but they must be very short commands, and preferably interrelated. You must also be aware that it may take you some time to formulate a phrase that feels just right. It has sometimes taken me as long as a week or more. Don't be impatient.

Once you have chosen your phrase and have got into an AT state in order to incorporate it, several, alternative, things may happen:

1   The phrase will feel good and comfortable, and you come out of your AT with it intact – that is, it will be the same at the end as at the beginning.
2   The phrase will feel awkward, and it will automatically change. Accept what comes up, and use it. Obviously, your unconscious and your conscious mind are more comfortable with the new format.
3   The whole concept may change while you are in your AT

state. This means that your unconscious mind's priority is different from your conscious perception. Respect your inner wisdom, and use the new phrase or concept that has come up.

To clarify this latter point, I will give you an example.

A trainee had joined one of my groups to use AT in order, ostensibly, to try to give up smoking. He chose the phrase 'Smoking gives me up', and went into his AT exercise in order to incorporate that phrase. He was smiling when he came out of his AT state. When I asked him what had gone on, he said that the phrase that had come up was 'I am calm and centred', which, of course, had nothing to do with smoking. But he then said, 'when I really think about it, this phrase makes much more sense, as I have just been made redundant and my marriage is on the rocks!' He used the phrase that had come up, and when I saw him a couple of months later and asked him how he had got on, he replied, 'Great! I have managed to get myself a new job, and am sorting my marriage out'. When I asked him about the smoking he replied, 'I'm still smoking, but I'm really enjoying it now!' However, he has since given up smoking, without having to use any particular phrases. As he sorted his life out, he said, he felt that he had no more need for smoking, and so it was quite easy for him to give it up.

This little episode demonstrates that this man's unconscious mind had a completely different agenda from his conscious perception. His unconscious mind showed him, while he was in his AT state, that this different agenda was far more important. Having taken heed of it, he was able to sort out his life.

If smoking is really your problem, you have to work out how you want to go about it. Some people like to make the cigarettes taste foul. Others like to say that they have no need for them. Yet others like to put the onus of giving up onto the cigarettes or the bad habit itself. (See page 265.)

As I mentioned earlier, positive affirmations are designed both to overcome, alter or modify the negative aspects of ourselves – the parts that we do not like or that hinder our progress towards a better quality of life – and to reaffirm the positive qualities that we already have but that we need to boost. To give you a taste of the wide range of sentences or phrases that you can utilise, I will cite a few examples. More will be given in the sections on specific conditions and situations discussed in Part 3 of this book. Obviously, the best ones are those that you make up yourself to suit your own personal needs.

We often need to pay special attention to particular situations, such as trying to lose weight, when you have to break it down into its various components, and work on the details in order to achieve your purpose. Let's take obesity as our example. Just to use the phrase 'I know I will lose weight' is inadequate. First of all, it projects the process into the future. Secondly, it does not indicate what may actually be causing the weight problem – eating too much at each meal, nibbling between meals, or eating the wrong foods. We assume, of course, that there is no underlying medical cause.

A better way of approaching the problem would be to try to analyse it, either by thinking about it yourself or by discussing it with a friend or counsellor. Am I eating too much at each meal? Do I pick in between meals? Do I eat too many fatty or sweet things? Do I eat too much because I am depressed, anxious or angry? And so on. Once you have sorted out what the basic problem is, then you can work on it. For instance, if the over-eating is due to depression or to other emotional problems, it is best to work at the offloading exercises as well as using a relevant affirmation formula. If it is due to any other reason, you can make up a specific formula for that particular problem. However, **it is extremely important to be absolutely honest with yourself and about the possible causes of your problems.** Unless you are honest and try to get to the bottom of things, you will not get very far.

Before giving a few sample phrases, it is worth mentioning another use to which the deep state of AT can be put. If you are looking for an answer to a puzzle or a problem, or if you want some inspiration about a specific subject, think hard about it before doing an AT exercise, and then forget about it while you are actually doing your AT. You may find that the answer to your problem, or the required inspiration, will appear when you get deeply into your AT state. Don't be impatient or expect anything, just think about it and yet remain passive about the whole thing. If anything happens, regard it as a great bonus. A lot of people, myself included, have had some of their best inspirations in that deep state of AT.

A few examples:

'I am calm and creative.'
'I love myself, life and living.'
'I love every new day, and the joy that it brings me.'
'I can go on living and loving, and nothing will deter me from that.'
'I know that my inner space is full of love, light, beauty and peace.'
'I am confident that I can overcome my disease (disability).'
'My life is full of love, light and joy, and there is no space for the disease.'
'The love and the serenity that I feel can dispel the disease.'
'I am a loving and lovable being, with important contributions to make to life (society [or whatever]).'
'I am strong, healthy, and full of energy.'
'I am full of energy and vitality.'
'I accept myself totally.'
'I am responsible for myself and my life.'
'I am calm and confident.'

More examples are given in the subject sections of Part 3. Do remember that the most important and effective ones are those that you make up yourself, for your own needs.

Lesson 10 The space exercise, advanced positive affirmations, and the healing-light meditation exercise

This lesson should only be used when you feel that you have mastered your AT properly and that you can go into deep states of relaxation. For most people, this usually means about two months after completing lesson 9, but this will obviously depend to a large extent on how diligently and regularly you have been practising the exercises since then. Most people find that by now they do not do their exercises three or more times a day, but it is important to do your full standard exercises (lessons 1 to 4 and 6 to 9) AT LEAST ONCE A DAY in order to help you remain calm and relaxed. The use of the exercises in this lesson is purely optional.

If you try to use this lesson before you are ready, you will not gain the benefits that you are seeking.

Lesson 10 is divided into three parts:

1 The introduction of the *space exercise*.
2 A more advanced use of *positive affirmations*.
3 The introduction of the *healing-light meditation exercise*.
(See also lesson 11.)

THE SPACE EXERCISE

There are three main uses for this exercise: (1) **on its own as a quick and effective exercise to get you relaxed**, particularly when you have no time or inclination to do any of the other exercises; (2) **as a means of deepening the AT state**, and hence its beneficial effects, even further; (3) **to cut down intruding thoughts**, if you happen to be particularly beset by them.

1 If you wish to use the space exercise on its own, you do it after the scan, and end with 'I am at peace' and then cancel.

2   If you wish to use it in order to deepen your AT state it is best to introduce it after 'My neck and shoulders are heavy' and before 'I am at peace'.

3   In order to reduce, or even banish, intruding thoughts, especially at the beginning of an AT exercise, the best point to introduce it is after your scan and before 'My right (left) arm is heavy'.

How do I do the space exercise?

It is almost like doing a reverse scan: start with your face, and work down your body to your feet. The phrase that we use is '**I imagine a space between my** (eyes, ears, etc.)'. (I will give more detail in a moment.) There are a number of ways of imagining this space, and you have to find the way that suits you best and that you feel most comfortable with. I'll mention a few that trainees have found useful, but remember that you may find a better way of doing it yourself.

Some people like to imagine that a blind or curtain is being pulled down in front of them, starting at the top of the head and gradually moving down the body, so that by the time they reach their feet they have completely disappeared behind the curtain. Others like to imagine that they are a glass container filled with a coloured liquid; as the mind drifts down the body, the container gradually empties, and by the time it reaches their feet they consist of an empty transparent container. Yet others prefer to imagine that the areas between the body parts that they focus on are wiped out and disappear: that is to say, when you say, 'I imagine a space between my shoulders and elbows', the whole of the area between the shoulders and the elbows on both sides (including the trunk in the middle) disappears. But if you use this technique, do make sure that you start from the outside of one limb and go the outside of the other one on the opposite side – otherwise, you'll end up with a space in the middle and the edges of your body dangling on the outside! This does you no harm, but can feel mighty peculiar! You may have to try each of the ways just described a number of times, in order to find the one that you feel most comfortable with.

It is best to try the exercise on its own initially, in order to see how you get on, before you introduce it as part of your full

AT exercise. Having decided how you want to imagine the space, proceed as follows:

1   *As an effective way to relax yourself:*

Get into a correct AT position.
Scan.
Take your attention to your face and eyes, and repeat each of the following phrases 2 or 3 times:

'I imagine a space between my eyes.'
'I imagine a space between my ears.'
'I imagine a space between my shoulders.'
'I imagine a space between my upper arms.'
'I imagine a space between my elbows.'
'I imagine a space between my forearms.'
'I imagine a space between my wrists.'
'I imagine a space between my hands.'
'I imagine a space between my hips.'
'I imagine a space between my thighs.'
'I imagine a space between my knees.'
'I imagine a space between my lower legs.'
'I imagine a space between my ankles.'
'I imagine a space between my feet.'
'I am at peace.'
Cancel.

Once you have mastered the technique of the exercise on its own, you can try ways 2 and 3:

2   *As a means of deepening the AT state:*

Get into position.
Scan.
'My right (left) arm is heavy.'
And so on through all the formulae learnt in lessons 1, 2, 3, 4, 6 and 7, repeating each one 2 or 3 times.
'My neck and shoulders are heavy.'
Do the space exercise as described on page 134 above.
'I am at peace.'
Cancel or repeat the exercise 2 or 3 times, depending on how long you want it to last.

3   *To reduce or banish intruding thoughts:*

Get into an AT position.
Scan.
Do the space exercise as described on page 134.
'My right (left) arm is heavy.'
'My arms and legs are heavy and warm.'
And so on until the end of the exercises, with all the formulae,
repeating each exercise 2 or 3 times.
'I am at peace.'
Cancel, or repeat the whole thing 2 or 3 times if you wish.

A MORE ADVANCED USE OF POSITIVE AFFIRMATIONS

Now that you can get deep into your healing space, you can
utilise it in order to support or reinforce the effects and
benefits that you have already gained by using the standard
exercises. Positive affirmations can also be used, in conjunction with the space exercise, to bring relief to certain parts of
the body: for example, to cool an itchy patch. It is of **para-**
mount importance that if you do have any persistent symptom
it is investigated and its cause determined. The advanced use of
the positive affirmations should not be a substitute for the
proper elucidation of the cause of any symptom or its proper
treatment. If you do have persistent symptoms, positive
affirmations should be used only in conjunction with other
methods of treatment, in order to enhance and reinforce their
effect by calling upon your own healing reserves. For instance, if you have a blockage in your bowel no amount of AT
will get rid of it. You must have it treated surgically. However, your AT and the positive affirmations will help you to
recover much more quickly. (See specific subject sections in
Part 3.)

There are **three situations in which you must not use**
advanced positive affirmations:

1   **Never use them to affect the heart.** The only reference to
the heart should be confined to 'My heartbeat is calm and
regular'.
2   **Never use them to affect your brain.** The nearest we get to
this is when we use the scalp – superficially – in the scan, and

when we use the phrase, 'My forehead is cool and clear'. You must, though, be aware that you are already indirectly affecting all the functions of your body, including your brain, when you use the standard exercises.

3   **Never use them to affect the sexual organs directly.** In one experiment, healthy medical students were asked to warm their testicles in their AT state. It was found that their sperm production diminished almost to nothing during the exercises, but returned to normal after they stopped warming them.

In accordance with autogenic training principles, to make up your own phrases for the advanced use of positive affirmations you use the same basic sensations as in the standard exercises: namely, heaviness, warmth, cooling. You also use 'it', as in the phrase, 'It sleeps me'. I give some examples below, but there are more in the subject sections in Part 3.

Once you have taken account of the important points above, you can use the power of the mind to help improve your condition. For instance, if you have an infected area on the back of your hand which is warm and painful, you can go through the following procedure. Get into your AT state, as usual. Once you are deep into it, direct your attention to the infected area and keep repeating the phrase that you have decided on: for example, 'The back of my hand is cool' – which seems the most appropriate. And introduce it where it feels right: perhaps after 'My arms and legs are heavy and warm', or after 'My forehead is cool and clear' – again, wherever feels most appropriate.

If you have an ache in your lower abdomen, for instance, use a phrase such as 'My lower abdomen is warm (heavy, cool)', depending on what feels right, and introduce it after 'My solar plexus is warm', as you are already in that vicinity. Or if you are suffering from a cold, try the following regime to help you get over it, or at least make your symptoms more bearable. Having got into a deep AT state, use this pattern of positive affirmations, introducing them after 'My forehead is cool and clear' and repeating them as often as you like:

'My eyes are cool and clear.'
'My nose is cool and clear (dry).'
'My throat is cool (warm).'

'My chest is warm' – to help your cough.
'My neck and shoulders are heavy.'
'I am at peace.'
Cancel.

You can use these affirmations as part of your full AT exercises 3 times a day. You can also use several abbreviated exercises, including affirmations, in order to reinforce the process of alleviating your symptoms. You can continue making up your own phrases, as appropriate. Here are a few examples:

'Warmth and comfort make me sleepy' – for sleeplessness.
'It sleeps me' – for sleeplessness.
'My fingers (toes, nose) are (is) warm' – for frostbite or circulation problems.
'My bottom (anus, vulva) is cool' – for itchy bottom or vulva.
'My eyes and eyelids are cool and clear' – for itchy eyes or hay fever.
'My throat is cool (warm)' – for sore throat.
'My breathing is calm and regular' – for asthma.

THE HEALING-LIGHT MEDITATION EXERCISE

Guided visualisation or *guided imagery* is a technique which is often used to utilise the hidden powers of the mind and body in order to try and deal with specific issues. Therefore, both the methods and the contents can be very variable (see Further Reading). I have found this particular one easy to follow and quite effective. Once it has been used a few times on its own, it can then be incorporated into the space exercise, either in its entirety, or just the part to do with changing lights and colours.

It is usually very difficult to imagine things at the same time as remaining passive in order to get into the exercise fully and derive the maximum benefit from it. In addition, this exercise is a long one, with many instructions. It is therefore best either to be taken through this exercise by someone else or to tape-record it and play it back to yourself. If you record it, make sure that you speak slowly, calmly and confidently, as this will make quite a difference to your mood and the way you feel about the exercise. It is also important to remember that not everyone *sees* things in their mind's eye. Some people feel the scene, some hear it, some smell it, and yet others use a combination. There is no right or wrong way of doing it, and all are absolutely fine. The most important thing is that you feel comfortable with it and that you use as many of your senses as possible.

Remember that this is a very powerful technique, and may bring you in touch with a great many powerful emotions, memories or feelings that need to be dealt with. Furthermore, when we use the word *healing* in this context we use it in the broadest possible sense; we include the resolution not only of physical problems but also of emotional, psychological or spiritual ones, present or past, latent or overt. **This meditation is designed to confuse the conscious, and to get directly into the unconscious.** By becoming incorporated into the unconscious the positive affirmations that are used with it become much more powerful. So don't worry if you lose track, become confused or cannot remember what has happened or what you were told. In fact it is at times when our conscious is confused in a deep state of relaxation that the door to the unconscious mind opens wider. The point is that you will have absorbed it all subliminally into your unconscious. It is also perfectly all right if you *can* follow and *can* remember everything. Our minds all work differently. But the fact is that, irrespective of how yours works, the end result will be as good as anyone else's. YOU WILL BENEFIT from this exercise.

How do I do it?

Get into a comfortable position, either sitting in an armchair or, preferably, lying down. Scan as usual, so that you feel completely relaxed and comfortable. If you do not feel particularly relaxed, you can do a quick AT before you start. The dashes (——) in the instructions that follow indicate that there should be a pause if you are recording or if someone is reading them to you. Having got into position and relaxed, proceed as follows:

Imagine yourself in some natural setting on a beautiful sunny day. Choose a place where you feel comfortable, confident and secure. It can be either imaginary or real: in a garden, in a meadow, by the sea or in the mountains – anywhere at all.

Having chosen your place, give yourself a few moments to fix the scene well into your mind.

Then **look around you slowly and deliberately**. Are there any plants about? —— Any shrubs? —— Any trees? —— Any flowers? —— **Look at the colours and the textures.** —— Feel the plants or anything else in the vicinity, if you wish. ——

Are there any smells? ——

Any sounds? —— Perhaps the sound of birds singing? —— Flowing water? —— Or a gentle rustle of the wind? —— Any other sounds? ——

You can feel the warmth of the sun on your body, and that makes you feel even more relaxed, content and happy. **Allow the rays of the sun to permeate you and, as they do so, feel any fear, anxiety or apprehension that you may have felt now dissipate through the warm glow of the sun's rays.**

You are now feeling extremely relaxed, comfortable, calm and confident.

If you are not already sitting down in your imaginary scene, find yourself a comfortable place and sit down. You may lie down if you wish. Look ahead into the beautiful blue sky and feel the warmth of the sun dissipating any remnants of self-doubt or unease that you may have felt.

Imagine the sun's rays breaking up into their various refractions and colours, shining on different parts of your body as I go through them:

Imagine a red light shining on the lower part of your body, starting with your feet and slowly extending along your calves and shins, thighs and lower stomach.

Feel the warmth of this wonderful healing light on the lower part of your body. Allow it to slowly and gently permeate you and, as it does so, feel its healing powers merge with your own healing powers, to dissolve any pain, distress or discomfort that you may be feeling in that part of your body, whether physical, emotional, psychological or spiritual.

Keep this healing light on your legs and the lower part of your stomach, and allow it to make you feel confident, content, peaceful and healed.

Now imagine a beautiful orange healing light shining on the upper part of your stomach. Feel the warmth and glow of this magnificent healing light permeating throughout your upper stomach and stimulating your own healing powers. Feel it dissolve your infection, growth or any other disease, disability or distress that you may be harbouring in your body.

Keep the red light on your legs and lower stomach. Keep the orange light on your upper stomach, and feel the tremendous surge of healing powers going through your body. Feel yourself become more relaxed, content, confident and healthy.

Now imagine a golden-yellow light on your chest and arms. Allow the warmth and glow of this beautiful healing light to shine all the way through you, and allow it to stimulate and merge with your own healing powers – that extraordinary abundance of self-healing powers that you have within yourself, and that you can use not only to heal yourself, but also to overcome any other troubles or difficulties that you may have in your life.

Keep the golden-yellow light on your chest; the red light on your legs and lower stomach; and the orange light on your upper stomach. Feel yourself getting more and more confident, content and happy. Feel yourself improving in your confidence in overcoming any disease, difficulty or discomfort from which you may be suffering.

Imagine a beautiful cool green healing light shining on your throat and face. Feel this beautiful healing light, in combination with all the others, help to stimulate your own healing powers and allow any disease, distress or discomfort, whether physical, emotional, psychological or spiritual, to dissolve away.

Keep the red light on your legs and lower stomach; the orange light on your upper stomach; the golden-yellow light on your chest and arms; and the cool green healing light on your throat and face.

Allow all these healing lights to trigger your own healing powers; and, together, to help you heal any disease, distress or discomfort in your body. Feel how comfortable, relaxed, confident and peaceful you are. You are now fully aware that you can overcome any difficulty or adversity, both now and in the future.

Now imagine a beam of healing blue light coming out of each eye and disappearing into infinity. This blue light will take out of your body any remaining disease, distress or discomfort that may still be present, and deposit it in infinity.

Keep the red light on your legs and lower stomach; the orange light on your upper stomach; the golden-yellow light on your chest and arms; the green on your throat and face.

Allow these wonderful healing lights to dissolve any disease, whether infectious, malignant or any other sort; and any distress, whether emotional, psychological or spiritual. Allow these dissolved remnants to be incorporated into the blue light and taken out of your being and deposited in infinity.

Now imagine a beautiful healing silver-white light enveloping your forehead and the top of your head. —— This most healing light of all will make total that healing which will have been started by the other lights. It will make you feel good, whole, complete and totally healed.

Now allow this magnificent silver-white light to gradually move down from your forehead and overtake all the other lights, which will dissolve in its wake as will any problems or distress that you may have felt before starting this guided imagery. Allow the silver-white light to come slowly down your face —— ; your neck —— ; your shoulders, chest and arms —— ; your stomach and pelvis —— ; and your legs —— .

You are now completely covered by this silver-white light —— ; this most healing of all lights —— . Allow yourself to merge into this light and become part of it, so that you can feel its wholeness, purity, freedom and ultimate healing powers – which are in fact your own healing powers, with which you are only just becoming familiar —— . Observe how wonderfully peaceful, content, happy and healed you feel at

this moment. These feelings will stay with you even after you have completed this journey.

Now allow some of this healing silver-white light to seep away from you and form a beautiful circle of silver light in front of you ——— . Feel your healing powers and energies extending to this circle of healing silver light in front of you.

Now imagine any one individual, or number of individuals, whom you wish to be healed with you in this circle of silver light ——— . Accept freely whoever or whatever (animal, bird or insect) comes into your circle.

(Allow at least one minute of silence at this point, so that you can both fix the people whom you wish to heal in the circle and have enough time to send them your healing energies, so that they can benefit from the ultimate power and energy of the healing light with which you are now in contact.)

Allow those in the circle to gently fade away, for they have already benefited from the tremendous powers of the healing energy – just as you yourself have.

You may find, once they have gone, that there is a gift left for you in the circle. This may be physical, emotional, psychological or spiritual, but you will recognise it for what it is. If there is a gift left for you, commit it to your memory, as you will be able to draw strength from it whenever in the future you are faced with difficulty, hardship or distress. All that you need to do is relax deeply and think of your gift.

Now allow the silver circle of light in front of you to gently disappear ——— . Allow the same thing to happen to the silver-white light that has been surrounding you, and gently bring your mind back to the present and to the room in which you started the exercise. Get ready to terminate the exercise.

As you move forward and start coming out of your guided imagery, remember that once you have come out of the exercise you will still feel confident, relaxed, content and at peace. You will be aware of the tremendous healing powers that you have within yourself, and which you can utilise at any time you wish. You will also have the confidence of being able to overcome any disease, difficulties or hardships that you may be faced with, now or in the future.

Now bring your attention fully to the present, and feel the hardness of the floor (chair or whatever, depending on your position) **beneath you. Feel yourself fully grounded, and cancel in the usual way.**

Remember that if you have gone very deeply into this guided imagery, as some people can, you may have to cancel several times. That does not matter, but DO ENSURE that you are well out of the state of AT and relaxation and that your reflexes are back to their normal sharpness by the time you want to continue with your normal routine.

In the context of this guided imagery or guided visualisation we refer to 'healing' in the broadest sense of the word and NOT necessarily in the sense of 'curing', although that may also happen from time to time. The healing may be as diverse as becoming able to deal with one's own present physical, emotional or spiritual problems, or with one's unresolved problems from the past, and may include unresolved problems in a relationship either now or in the past. It may even involve the healing of unresolved emotions with someone who is dead. The best example of this that I can think of concerns one of my trainees with AIDS.

I had done several of these *healing meditations* with him, and both the images and the people whom he wished to be healed with him in the circle of light were always different. On one occasion he was crying when he came out of the meditation. He said that the picture that had come to his mind was of his mother, who had been dead for about four years. She was dancing and twirling in the centre of the circle. Eventually he joined her, and they danced together until they merged into one. He found this extremely moving, because he felt that at last he had managed to resolve a lot of unresolved feelings, including the anger that had poisoned their relationship before her death. He was very thankful that he had managed to heal the rift between them, which had soured his feelings for her for so long.

Don't worry if there do not seem to be any gifts left for you at the end of the exercise, if no obvious healing seems to have happened, or if you do not understand the nature or the meaning of the gift left for you in the circle. The healing may occur at an unconscious level, and sometimes the end result can only be seen over the longer term, or after a succession of imagery trips.

In order to explain these points further, I'll give another example. What I am going to describe happened to a person with AIDS, with whom I had worked a great deal.

In one of his AT states he came up with the spontaneous image of a red-hot coal fire. He had the feeling that this symbol was quite important as far as his healing processes were concerned. We tried to think of all the hot things that he could indulge in, such as saunas or eating hot curries. He even thought of rolling in a bed of nettles, which I did not think was a good idea! We drew a blank for the time being, as he felt that none of the suggestions had the right feel about them. Months later, while he was in New York, quite by chance he came across a workshop that dealt, among other things, with walking on fire. He immediately felt that that fitted his AT image of months earlier. He attended the workshop, and managed to walk over about ten feet of red-hot coals without getting as much as a blister! He was confident that that was exactly the feeling he had had in his spontaneous visualisation.

He felt wonderful after the fire walk, and he also felt that he had reached a watershed in his fight to conquer AIDS. This demonstrates that sometimes you have to wait quite a while for the interpretation of what you observed during your AT state. It also shows that each person's visualisations are absolutely unique to him or her, and that they will vary from time to time, depending on circumstances and on the stage of development and growth of the individual.

Lesson 11 Autogenic meditation

There is nothing very special about the term, and don't let yourself be put off by the possible esoteric associations of the word *meditation*. All that it alludes to here is the very deep state that follows the standard AT exercises, some manifestations of which, such as the spontaneous appearance of colour, have already been mentioned. Unfortunately, at present we have no other term for it. There are **six stages**, or exercises, that you can undertake in order to reach this deep state, during which – apart from feeling very relaxed and comfortable – you will find yourself able to achieve any specific goals that you may like to set yourself. These stages can be worked through either individually or together, depending on your needs and inclinations.

The beginnings of *autogenic meditation* seem to flow naturally from the practice of the standard exercises, and this is why the exercises that we are about to explore now are sometimes called *second-stage autogenics*. As in standard AT, this stage, also, trains you in a particular type of PROCEDURE. It teaches you a WAY in which both mind and body can get on with the very personal task of improving your physical, emotional and spiritual health and well-being. There are no prescribed values, beliefs or insights associated with the practice of autogenic meditation. Whatever does or does not happen is highly individualistic, and absolutely impossible to predict. Having said that, you can be sure that you will find it enjoyable and valuable – depending on how much you put into it.

AUTOGENIC MEDITATION: THE SIX STAGES

1   *The spontaneous evocation of colours*
(colour meditation)

You will know that you are ready for this stage if you are
already seeing colours spontaneously during your standard
AT exercises, or if you can sustain a calm, and almost
undisturbed, standard exercise for almost half an hour.

Having done a good standard AT exercise, stay in that state
without cancelling. You may eventually find that you become
aware of a colour or light which seems as if projected onto the
inner 'screen' of your closed eyelids. When that happens,
don't try to actively follow it, for if you do, you are bound to
lose your colours as well as your truly passive AT state. The
appearance of colour can take a few minutes or half an hour.
Remember that it can take a few days of practising AT before
colours start appearing.

I mentioned earlier that there are a number of different
ways that the colours (or lights) may present themselves. You
may become aware of squares of different colours, or of
star-bursts such as you get with fireworks, or swirls of multi-
coloured haze or smoke. Or you may see colours in entirely
different ways, that are specific to you. Whatever the presen-
tation, you will find that as you **passively** observe them and
allow them to develop they will eventually merge into one,
and a single colour or light will completely fill your visual
field. It is a very enriching, fulfilling and healing moment
when this happens, and whatever colour you see at this point
will be your *base colour*. You will find that whenever you get
deeply relaxed, that colour will spontaneously appear.
Colours can take anything from a few days to a few weeks to
appear. But once you get the knack, you will find that your
colour can appear very rapidly – even during your space
exercise, which is very rewarding.

**A word of warning: if the colour red coupled with a sense of
aggression or violence intrudes and dominates, cancel
immediately.** If the same thing happens on more than two
occasions in quick succession, it is best to leave your colour

meditation for a while and concentrate on offloading the uncomfortable feelings that are presenting themselves (lesson 5). However, if the colour red, even if associated with feelings of moderate anger, appears only occasionally and is not too distressing, then you can go on with your meditation, in conjunction with the offloading exercises. You will find that eventually you will be able to work through the disharmony that is obviously present.

At the end of your colour meditation, which may last 10 to 15 minutes, cancel as usual. The whole exercise usually takes between 45 minutes and an hour.

SUMMARY

Get into a correct AT position.
Scan.
Do an AT exercise.
Maintain your passive state of mind for about 30 minutes.
Allow colours or lights to develop and passively observe them for 10–15 minutes.
Cancel.

Remember that there is no fixed length of time for doing each of the stages. Just move on to the next one when you feel that you are ready to do so.

2 The evocation of colours on demand

Once you have found your own base colour, you are ready to move on to the next stage. At this point, start to think of specific colours **actively** in your AT state, and watch what happens and what associations come up. It is best to try a few different colours in each meditation, and to finish the exercise with your own base colour.

SUMMARY

Get into an AT position.
Scan.
Do an AT exercise.
Maintain your passive state of mind for about 30 minutes.

Think of specific colours, observe what form each colour or light takes, and what feelings, emotions or memories may be associated with each colour. Think of your own base colour, and stay in that colour for as long as you wish.
Cancel.

3 *Visualising objects*

Once you can achieve the appearance of colours on demand, you are ready to move on to this phase. Start imagining concrete objects, such as a vase, a tea-cup, a flower or fruit, one at a time, and once they have taken shape in your mind try to experience them in their entirety, using all your senses: vision, hearing, touch, smell and taste. Try to experience several objects in each of your meditations. Do remember, though, that although you are supposed to be visualising objects rather than colours, you may find by this stage that you will slip into a colour mood very quickly. If that happens, imagine the object against a background of the colour that seems to be prevalent.

SUMMARY

Get into an AT position.
Scan.
Do an AT exercise and maintain the passive state for about 30 minutes.
Visualise concrete objects, and experience them with all your senses.
Cancel.

4 *Visualising a person*

This stage is very similar to the last one, but instead of an object you imagine a person. It is best to start imagining people whom you know reasonably well but with whom you are not too emotionally involved. Once you can manage that, you can move on to visualising people you are more intimately associated with. Once you have fixed him or her in your mind, passively watch to see what sorts of feelings, emotions and memories come up. You may be able to resolve any difficulties that you have in your relationship with this particular person. You may think of specific questions to do with him or her, to which you want answers. You may be surprised at the number of revelations that come up in this state, and that enable you to deal with unresolved problems in your relationship with the other person.

SUMMARY

Get into an AT position.
Scan.
Do an AT exercise and maintain your passive state for about 30 minutes.
Visualise different people, and try to experience them in their totality.
Cancel.

5 *The imaginative evocation of concepts*

Once you have got into an AT state and maintained it for a while, start thinking about abstract words, concepts or emotions such as forgiveness, love, peace, anger, freedom, prejudice and so on. Either wait for them to come up spontaneously, or think of specific subjects that you wish to work on. The important thing to note is that once you have thought of a word you must sit back **passively** and watch what happens. You may get in touch with certain feelings, or you may start seeing pictures, images or symbols. Accept whatever form the concept presents itself in, and allow it complete freedom to go the way it wants to. The only time that you should terminate the exercise prematurely by cancelling is if you get in touch with a lot of powerful or uncomfortable emotions. If this happens, you will need to work on them, using the offloading exercises (lesson 5).

SUMMARY

Get into a correct AT position.
Scan.
Do an AT exercise and maintain the state of passive concentration for about 30 minutes.

Think of abstract words, concepts or emotions that you want to work on.
Cancel when you are ready.

6 *Using self-directed questions*

In this final stage you are using your AT state to try to gain more information about yourself, and to find answers and solutions to your queries and problems. This procedure was introduced when you learned how to use positive affirmations in a more advanced way (page 135).

What you do here is get into a deep AT state, start thinking of sentences that are appropriate to you and your circumstances, and then sit back passively and watch what happens. Before you start your AT, think hard about the questions that you want to work on, as it is sometimes quite difficult to think of a relevant question while you are in a deep state, unless it comes up spontaneously. In some instances, though, this is exactly what you want. Don't forget that you can use a combination of thought-out *and* spontaneous questions. And you can work on more than one question at a time, especially if they are closely related.

I often use this technique if I am stuck for inspiration when I am writing, or when I want to work on a specific part of myself and my personality. The way I usually do it is to think hard, before my AT, about the subject that I want to write about, and then get into a prolonged AT state, and just sit back and see what happens. Sometimes I get the answer in that very session, but more often than not it pops up spontaneously in one of my later ATs or in my dreams. The questions that one can deal with in this way are, of course, limitless and highly individualistic, as they spring from one's current needs or problems.

SUMMARY

Get into a correct position.
Scan.
Do an AT exercise, and maintain the passive state for about 30 minutes.
Think of a question that you wish to work on.

Allow it to develop as it wants to while you remain totally passive about it.
Cancel when you are ready.

It is very important to remember that once you have mastered the technique of autogenic meditation you can either use each stage separately or combine any number together. You will also find that in time you will be able to get into the meditative state very quickly, at the end of a normal AT exercise, especially when you are using the space exercise. So you will be able to draw on its tremendous benefits whenever you like.

PART 3

Conditions and activities where AT can be of help

§11 How do I use Part 3?

You can read Part 3 straight through, or you can use it like a reference book. It covers fifty-one conditions and activities that can be helped by the practice of AT. As you look through the pages that follow, you will discover that autogenic training is used not only *to prevent, manage and treat a whole range of medical conditions, diseases and disabilities, but also as a tool for improving performance and enhancing enjoyment in a great variety of other fields, such as acting and sport, education and industry.*

It is important to note, though, that the list of activities and conditions given here is by no means exhaustive. There are others, both medical and non-clinical, which lie outside the scope of this book. But even if your own special requirements are not covered here, you may still find autogenic training useful when it comes to managing your personal situation, provided that you take into account the comments made in §8, on precautions. If it is at all possible, though, do discuss your special needs with a qualified trainer.

Bear in mind that the comments and statements made in Part 3 are no more than a guide, as unfortunately space does not permit us to go into each subject in great detail. However, those of you who are interested in studying any topic in greater detail will find the Appendices and Further Reading list useful.

It must also be appreciated that I have not mentioned every therapy that might be useful in each condition specified. This would have inevitably introduced too much repetition; and furthermore, certain therapies, such as iridology (mainly used as a diagnostic tool), homoeopathy and Chinese and Indian herbal medicine, tend to treat clusters of symptoms in the context of the individual whole person, and that makes it very difficult to fit them into the kind of medical classification system normally used to describe diseases in standard

Western medicine. *Spiritual healing* (or faith and contact healing) also falls into this category, as the whole purpose seems to be directed towards enabling and empowering the individual while supporting him. So if you feel that a certain complementary therapy might be of benefit to you, or if you are just curious to find out more about any of those mentioned, it would be well worth your while to contact the headquarters for that particular therapy or an organisation associated with it (details are given in the Appendices), who would be delighted to supply you with further information.

§12 Acting

Acting is a very stressful and precarious job, except for a small number of successful individuals. The stress and the resultant anxiety are not just confined to the times when the actor is working: they also affect the periods in between jobs, euphemistically called 'resting'. For far from resting, he or she is faced with enormous stresses – financial and social, as well as having constantly to attend auditions. Then, while an actor is working, there is the continual strain of appearing in front of audiences and cameras, of having to memorise scripts, of travelling and staying in strange and sometimes uncomfortable situations and settings.

The *standard AT exercises* have been found to be extremely helpful not only in controlling and dealing with these various stresses, but also in *improving concentration and the ability to memorise scripts*. By doing a full set of AT exercises before going on stage or on camera, actors find that they can perform much more effectively and competently. They can also use the phrase 'My neck and shoulders are heavy' as a *partial exercise* while acting, in order to control their stress levels and keep themselves calm and confident. This enables them to remember their lines much more easily as well as to deliver them more effectively and powerfully, as they are not inhibited by tension and anxiety, which can make them freeze. However, this does *not* mean that they lose the adrenalin buzz which is essential for some individuals; they learn to use it advantageously. The *offloading exercises* (lesson 5) can also be of immense value in ridding various parts of the body of unwanted stresses, tensions and emotions.

The *positive affirmations* (lesson 9) can be used to alleviate specific problems, such as lack of confidence. There are numerous other ways, discussed elsewhere in Part 3 as well as in Part 2, in which AT can be useful to actors.

§13 AIDS

I dedicate this section and all my work in the field of autogenic training and serious disease and disability, especially HIV infection and AIDS, to all those who are fighting their condition, for their courage has been the main source of inspiration in my own work; and to those who have died, especially Peter and Tony, for in death we truly live on in the hearts, minds and memories of those who go on living. Those of us privileged to have known such individuals necessarily become the custodians of their unfulfilled dreams, hopes and aspirations. We owe it to them to go on fighting and to become the torch-bearers of hope and optimism, especially at times of darkness, doubt and confusion, when we ourselves risk losing direction.

AIDS, or acquired immune deficiency syndrome, is believed to be caused by the human immunodeficiency virus (HIV). This virus is quite delicate and does not survive outside the body for any length of time. It is caught only by the transfer of body fluids – blood, semen, vaginal secretions and possibly mother's milk – between two individuals in close contact. The transfer by mother's milk is still somewhat controversial. The virus is unlikely to be passed on through saliva. In most Western countries blood and blood products are now specially treated, and so catching HIV infection via blood transfusions and blood products is unlikely. However, direct blood contact still occurs between drug abusers, and so those who share needles can pass the infection to each other. It is therefore imperative to try to avoid drug abuse, and especially the sharing of needles.

The commonest means of spreading the disease is through unprotected penetrative sexual intercourse between two individuals. This can be sex between a man and a woman, or between two men. Contrary to earlier popular belief, the virus does not pick specific types of sexual partner. It can infect anyone who comes across it in sexual intercourse. So it is to be recommended that anyone who has multiple partners, or who has sex with a casual partner, avoids penetrative sex. If that is not possible, **it is extremely important for the man to use a condom** (sheath), in order to prevent the spread of AIDS, as this is the only way so far discovered of fighting this twentieth-century scourge. Only a few isolated cases of babies becoming infected through their mother's milk have been reported.

NEITHER HIV INFECTION NOR AIDS CAN BE PASSED ON BY EVERYDAY SOCIAL CONTACT SUCH AS TOUCHING OR KISSING, OR BY USING THE SAME CUPS OR GLASSES AS AN INFECTED PERSON, SO IT IS PERFECTLY ALL RIGHT TO CARRY ON ABSOLUTELY NORMALLY WHEN DEALING WITH ANYONE WHO IS HIV-INFECTED, SO LONG AS ONE DOES NOT COME INTO DIRECT CONTACT WITH HIS OR HER BODY FLUIDS.

The use of *autogenic training* as part of the holistic management of AIDS is very recent. I first undertook it in October 1985, with some unexpectedly good results from the point of view both of improving the quality and of prolonging the life of people with AIDS (PWAs). However, before going on to describe how AT has been used with PWAs, it is important to consider certain other aspects of the condition that are similar to those of other serious illnesses, as well as other factors, especially society's attitude, which seem to be peculiar to this disease. Indeed, society's attitude to AIDS makes the task of both the PWAs, who are fighting for their lives, and those caring for them, even more difficult than it needs to be.

In this day of bigotry and prejudice, in certain sections of our community more than others, it has been very easy to get onto the bandwagon of self-righteous indignation and dismiss those suffering from the infection as outcasts or as subhuman. Not least of all because the earliest cases reported in the West happen to have occurred amongst the Haitians, male homosexuals and intravenous drug abusers. I have come across no other disease that creates such negativity, outright hostility and rejection, even within the medical profession. I believe that the main reason for this, apart from ignorance, is the fact that no other disease makes us face the complexities, difficulties and ambivalence inherent in our own sexuality, morality and religious beliefs, as well as our fears of dying and of death, especially if it should threaten at a relatively young age. Those of us who have the privilege of being in the caring role – which, after all, includes almost everyone to some degree – must address all these points and be aware of our own feelings and reactions to them. It is imperative that we leave behind any prejudices that we may have, and that we do not bring them along to the bedside of a seriously ill or dying person; for they have enough burdens of their own to carry.

Furthermore, in this world of technological wizardry it is so easy for us as doctors to hide behind our computers, investigation results, prescription pads and bland denials, and lose sight of what caring is all about: the love, the compassion and the very act of being there, which are all of paramount importance in enabling the sick to come to terms with themselves and their disease and to empower themselves to rise above their disability and proceed along the road to healing.

The eight-week holistic courses run by me and my associates for HIV-positive people are fundamentally the same as those for any other group, and certainly the basic teaching of autogenic training is the same. But in my own groups I hope to act as a guide, to point out and illuminate the various paths that may be available, perhaps to be beaten down, in the jungle of both their internal and external worlds. At the same time to act as a mirror and reflect back all the love, kindness, compassion, dignity, peace, strength and, most of all, courage that lie deep within each one of them. Unfortunately, a lot of HIV-positive people are either unaware of these wonderful qualities within themselves or have allowed their inner light to be dimmed by feelings of self-doubt, guilt, shame, inadequacy and worthlessness, which are all too readily reinforced and exploited by current attitudes. During the course I hope to enable them to sweep away their negative feelings, so that once again that inner light can shine through.

As Pasteur, the French microbiologist, said rather simplistically, 'The bacteria are nothing; the terrain is everything'. In this case substitute virus for bacteria. For terrain, read all the many aspects of the body – mind – emotions – spirit equation. My aim is simple: it is to improve the terrain as much as possible, so that all treatment, whether based in orthodox medicine or in any of the complementary techniques, will have the best chance of being maximally effective. (These points have already been discussed in §5.)

It is important to pay particular attention to *diet* and *nutritional supplements*, and to *guided visualisations* and *positive affirmations*; and to reinforce the self-regulatory and healing processes that have already been triggered by practising autogenic training. It is also important that the affirmations should be gentle, passive and healing, and thus in keeping with the whole concept of autogenic training. Phrases such as 'I know I am healing myself' are very suitable. Aggressive and destructive visualisations, such as imagining sharks destroying the virus in the white cells, should be avoided, as that can lead to the reduction of the all-important T cells. These are a small sub-group of the white blood cells (CD4) which are essential for the defence of the body against infective organisms.

There are now some conventional medications which seem, at least, to arrest the destructive effects of the virus within the body. I tend to advocate other complementary therapies in addition to the individual's standard therapy. These include homoeopathy, herbal medicine and acupuncture, spiritual healing and reflexology (see Appendix 1), particularly for the control of some of the more troublesome symptoms, though a lot of these, such as weight loss, diarrhoea, night sweats and pain, can be controlled by the regular practice of autogenic training on its own. There has been at least one instance of someone managing to get rid of his skin cancer (Kaposi's sarcoma) lesions, using autogenic training and, in particular, *guided visualisations*; and another whose extensive glandular cancers regressed and who, by using AT in combination with radio- and chemotherapy, went into total remission. It is .interesting that the cancer had seemed to be totally unresponsive to the conventional therapies before he started doing AT. I also tend to advocate psychotherapy, counselling, co-counselling, creative art, music, dance (meditative or ordinary) – in fact, anything at all that enables an individual to get in touch with the tremendous healing powers that lie deep within himself.

Research by the author in 1994–5 showed that using a

combination of spiritual healing and AT, or of spiritual
healing and meditation, as part of holistic management of the
condition, **improved the CD4 count (T cells) of 85 per cent of
those attending by an average of 50 per cent** after four to eight
sessions of healing.

I feel that the most important contribution that we, as
carers, can make to prevent the dimming, even the ex-
tinguishing, of that beautiful life-flame in those who are
HIV-positive or have AIDS – while helping them to maintain
their well-being and improvement, and even go into remission – is to give them that CHANCE, that HOPE, that CONFIDENCE
that there is indeed an enormous reservoir of untapped
resources within themselves that they can fall back on in their
fight not only for survival, but also for a richer, fuller and
more meaningful life. For unless we have hope, unless we
have a purpose, a goal or an aspiration, and unless we have
faith in ourselves and our future, there is little left to live or
fight for. And fight they must, against an enemy whose main
weapon is the war of attrition that it wages against all aspects
of their being.

I believe that, with guidance and help, those with the HIV
infection or AIDS can become masters of their own destinies
rather than helpless victims of the disease. This can be
achieved by looking after all aspects of their bodies, minds,
emotions and spirit; and by becoming aware of and accepting
all the conflicts and paradoxes in their personalities, the
negative as well as the positive. By so doing they can make
contact with their inner strength and power, and develop
hope and confidence in themselves and their unbounding
capabilities. At that point they will begin to fully perceive
their potential, be able to rise above the paralysing and
destructive fear of disease and death, and proceed proudly
towards a much richer life, with all the love, beauty, peace,
contentment and fulfilment that it will bring – an experience
that can only be dreamed of by those who have never suffered
hardship, serious disability or a potentially fatal disease.

I also strongly believe that, whether we suffer from AIDS,
cancer or some other serious disease or disability – or, indeed,
are completely healthy – we can all achieve our ultimate aim
and ambition provided that we have enough belief in
ourselves and our capabilities and set our sights high enough,

accepting ourselves as the unique, whole, lovable and loving
individuals that in fact we are. Above all, we must strive
towards our ultimate goal, whatever it may be.

I hope that by the time my trainees have completed their
journey with me they will be able to cut through the oppressive bonds of negativity that confine them and move forward
into the light once again, with their minds full of constructive,
creative and positive thoughts; with their arms outstretched
to embrace all the unconditional love of their fellow-beings,
which could be an enormous source of power and energy in
their fight; and with their hearts full of hope, joy and laughter.
For despite all the heartache, hardship and hostility that they
encounter daily, life is still a miraculous thing, to be cherished
and enjoyed.

The figures for those with HIV infection and AIDS who
started attending my groups in late 1985 are as follows (these
are the updated figures that were available in December 1995).
Of the 14 people with advanced AIDS, the last died in 1994,
12 years after his diagnosis, the rest having an average
survival of four years, which is considerably better than
expected according to the majority of the statistics. Two of
those with ARC (AIDS related complex) have gone on to
AIDS and died. Two of those with PGL (persistent general-
ised lymphadenopathy) are doing well, and three out of the 14
HIV infected individuals with no symptoms have gone on to
develop full-blown AIDS (20.9 per cent). However, the most
striking finding in everyone who took part in the courses was
the fact that their quality of life improved considerably
following the completion of their training. Those who did
develop further complications found that they could not only
cope with the recurrences much more effectively, but also
recovered more quickly than expected.

These figures, especially those relating to people with
AIDS, confirm that stress management through the use of
autogenic training, together with attention to other aspects of
the individuals' lives, as well as the use of complementary
therapies in conjunction with conventional treatment, certainly leads not only to the prolongation of life, but more
importantly to the improvement of its quality.

§14   Angina (chest pain)

Here we shall concentrate on the chest pain that results from a reduction in the flow of blood to the heart and is usually known as angina. The chest pain associated with the heart usually comes on after exertion. To trigger an attack, this only needs to be minimal if the condition is very severe; the pain is relieved by rest. There are numerous other causes of chest pain, which I am not going to cover here. **It is therefore extremely important to have the cause of your chest pain established before you proceed any further.**

What can I do?

Autogenic training is particularly helpful for those who suffer from 'cardiac neurosis': that is to say, those who, in spite of having no underlying heart disease, have a morbid fear of having a heart attack; and those who have already had a heart attack and yet who, although their condition has resolved itself satisfactorily, are terrified of having another one. The most important thing, of course, is to try to prevent angina from developing in the first place, by following the advice given below and in §6. BUT ONCE THE DIAGNOSIS OF ANGINA IS MADE, YOU WILL BE ABLE TO DO A LOT TO RELIEVE THIS UNCOMFORTABLE CONDITION FOR YOURSELF.

Diet is very important, and you must avoid fried and other fatty foods, especially animal fats. Vegetable oils are much healthier for use in cooking, salad dressings and so on. Caffeine is detrimental to health, so try to avoid coffee, tea and other caffeine-containing drinks. Also, avoid red meats, as they are usually much fattier than white meats such as chicken and fish. Increase your intake of fibre, fresh fruit, vegetables and supplements, especially vitamins C and E, high dose magnesium, zinc, selenium, nicotinic acid, calcium, Omega 3 and 6 fatty acids (in fish oils, green vegetables especially lettuce, cabbage and spinach, walnuts, pecan nuts and linseed oil capsules) and lecithin (phosphodyl choline) which has been reported to dissolve the coronary blockages in a few cases.

Exercise is excellent, but you must keep within your own capabilities. Even if you can only manage a few minutes' walk, a gentle paddle in the swimming pool or just a few deep breaths and stretches, it will help to improve your circulation and general feeling of well-being. Try to work less hard. Take life more easily. Have plenty of leisure activities, and take regular holidays. Aim to reduce your stress levels in every aspect of your life. *Lose weight* if you are overweight.

There are, of course, *herbal, homoeopathic and conventional medications* that can help to relieve angina.

Autogenic training has an important role to play in the long-term management of this chronic condition. By reducing both blood pressure and blood cholesterol, which is known to be a very important factor in causing heart problems, AT can help to prevent angina from developing in the first place. Another of AT's important contributions is its ability to reduce stress and its effects. AT is also useful when the condition has become established. For it increases the blood flow to the heart and consequently increases the oxygen supply, thereby limiting the occurrence and the severity of the anginal attacks.

But before proceeding to use AT for this purpose, there are one or two **precautions** that you need to observe. **Firstly**, in rare instances it may actually aggravate the symptoms. If it does, obviously it means that AT is not right for you and your condition. **So don't use it.** The only way that you can find this out is by trying it, bearing in mind that you can cancel at once if you experience any unpleasant sensations. The majority of people with angina find AT beneficial, but if you have any doubts, only practise it initially under the guidance of a qualified trainer. **Secondly**, you may initially find it more comfortable to do AT in the sitting positions, then gradually introducing the lying-down posture. **Thirdly**, the use of 'My heartbeat is calm and regular' can trigger a certain amount of anxiety, particularly if there is already a strong element of fear associated with angina itself. In this situation it is best to leave the phrase out altogether, or introduce it very gradually. (See lesson 4 for further details.)

Having taken account of these precautions, you can use the *standard exercises*. You will find them very helpful in alleviating your symptoms. The *offloading exercises*, particularly those dealing with anger, frustration and anxiety, can also be very useful. But the most important thing to remember is that you may have to modify them considerably and do them more gently, reducing the degree of physical exertion that some of them call for, so that they do not trigger an angina attack.

Do not experiment with the positive affirmations for this condition. The only ones that you can try are:

'My heartbeat is calm and easy (comfortable).'
'My chest is warm.'
'My heart is gently warm.'

Feel free to use visualisations to 'see' or imagine the blockages in the coronary arteries clearing away when you are in a deep state of AT. (See visualisation and imagery in Endacott, M., *Encyclopaedia of Complementary Therapies* – details in Further Reading.)

§15 Anxiety

Anxiety and depression together are responsible for a very large proportion of the workload of a general practitioner. They cause an enormous amount of distress and hardship – not only to the sufferers but also to those close to them. This can lead to a great deal of morbidity, unhappiness and strife in the community as a whole. No group is immune from the upsetting effects of anxiety and depression. They can affect anyone at any time, especially when the stresses of everyday living and of relationships become overwhelming. Not even children are immune – indeed, anxiety and depression are particularly prevalent during the teens, as well as in old age.

Anxiety is, of course, a perfectly natural feeling that we all experience; it is an essential part of everyday living. The symptoms associated with it are usually due to the sympathetic release of the chemicals adrenalin or noradrenalin by the adrenal glands (see §1), and include an increase in the rate and strength of the heartbeat. This makes the individual aware of his heartbeat, perhaps for the first time, which can be very worrying (see pages 80, 92). It may become particularly noticeable when we are relaxing or in bed, especially when we lie with one ear against the pillow. There is also an increase in the breathing rate, and we may have cold, sweaty hands, butterflies in the stomach or even feelings of nausea which may lead to actual vomiting.

Everyone who is subjected to any form of stimulation, whether it be stressful and uncomfortable or exciting and/or pleasurable, experiences one or more of these symptoms. It is our perception which determines whether or not we feel anxious or stressed, excited or exhilarated. ONLY when the symptoms become persistent, uncomfortable or overwhelming are we said to be suffering from 'anxiety'. A racing driver, for instance, or a sportsman or an actor, find the adrenalin release prior to their performance thrilling and exciting, whereas most other people would find these activities nerve-racking and hence uncomfortable and stressful.

As mentioned in §1, the effects of adrenalin stimulation seem to be cumulative, and although one stressful situation may not cause us too much distress or discomfort, a concatenation of events may lead to trouble. Then it may require only one more little incident to tip us over into a state of anxiety – the proverbial last straw that breaks the camel's back. It is this accumulation of stressful events that fixes us in a state of continuous and persistent adrenalin production, with all its manifold symptoms. We become like a car that is being driven with the choke out all the time. This causes a continual overconsumption of petrol, leading in the end to engine failure. Similarly, when we are stuck in the fight-flight vicious circle of anxiety and stress, we use so much energy that we are left with very little to spare, and finish up feeling totally exhausted. In this situation we do not usually have much energy left for doing anything, even if on a conscious level we desperately went to. THE FACT THAT THE BODY'S ENERGY IS BURNT OUT ON AN UNCONSCIOUS LEVEL IS ONE OF THE MAIN REASONS WHY TIREDNESS AND EXHAUSTION ARE SUCH COMMON SYMPTOMS OF ANXIETY AND STRESS; in fact, they can be the only presenting symptoms. One of the characteristics of this kind of tiredness is that it is not relieved by any amount of rest or sleep. In fact, oversleeping seems to aggravate the situation.

However, it is important to remember that if you do suffer from severe and prolonged tiredness you should not automatically put it down to plain anxiety without first having it fully investigated. There could well be a physical cause. Indeed, most doctors would only put such tiredness down to stress and anxiety after exhaustive investigations fail to demonstrate any obvious physical cause.

The symptoms of anxiety are many and varied: they include restlessness, frustration, unhappiness, loss of concentration, irritability, nervousness, decreased appetite, weight loss, sleeplessness, troubled dreams, exhaustion despite plenty of sleep, headaches, dizziness, blackouts, weakness, feelings of breathlessness, hyperventilation, palpitations, disturbed bowel and urinary function and nausea. This is by no means a complete list, as a lot of the symptoms of anxiety are very subjective and individualistic. So you may have some special symptoms of your own.

It was thought, when the more modern tranquillisers became available, that here was the answer to the problem of anxiety. However, it has relatively recently been found that they themselves can cause addiction and both physical and psychological habituation. In some instances they can cause feelings of rage and the actual exacerbation of anxiety symptoms. Although it may be absolutely necessary for you to take them for a short time to help you over an immediate crisis, **tranquillisers should not be taken over a prolonged period.** The exception to this rule is that certain tranquillisers have other qualities, such as causing certain muscles to relax, and so may have to be taken for long periods by individuals with specific conditions that call for muscle relaxation. Such cases are few and far between, though, and anyone needing to take tranquillisers for this purpose should anyway be under the regular supervision of a doctor. In most cases the use of tranquillisers over a prolonged period cannot be justified. There are other ways of dealing with anxiety and its symptoms, which I shall discuss in a moment.

The other common addictive chemical that a great many people fall back on in order to cope with their stress and anxiety is, of course, alcohol. The unfortunate thing is that the onset of addiction is very slow and insidious, and usually by the time a person becomes aware of it he or she is well and truly hooked. That awareness, and the social implications of alcoholism, are often a source of additional stress and anxiety for the addict and for his or her family and friends.

What can I do to help myself?

The first thing to do is to try to OUTLINE THE MAIN TROUBLESOME SYMPTOMS, AS WELL AS THE CAUSES OF THE ANXIETY, by making a list like that discussed on page 92. Often, just by doing that and thus becoming aware of the causes of our anxiety, we can reduce it by as much as 70 per cent, simply by avoiding or circumventing the people, situations and so on that make us anxious, until we have become more proficient at dealing with the causes. These measures may be necessary to enable us to deal with our anxiety which may initially be overwhelming, until we have learnt the relaxation technique properly. Other things that we can do include *avoiding drinks with caffeine in them* such as coffee and strong tea, and certain soft drinks, as they can aggravate the symptoms. Drink plenty of *herbal teas*, some of which – including camomile and comfrey, which you may be able to find, together with less common ones, in your local healthfood shop – are known to have calming effects. You may also be able to find homoeopathic and herbal materials that will help you with your relaxation. **Do not depend on alcoholic drinks** to soothe your jangled nerves, as they can be even more addictive than tranquillisers (see above). Improve your *diet*, and take enough *nutritional supplements* (§6), especially if loss of appetite is one of your main symptoms. Remember that *massage* and other forms of *touch therapy* (for example, reflexology), *osteopathy* and *chiropractic* (see Appendices) can all help enormously, especially if you carry a lot of your tensions in your muscles.

Another possible way of reducing the level of your anxiety is to talk about the causes with a good friend, a counsellor, a therapist, a priest or some other religious leader. This may enlarge your spiritual dimension at the same time. You may find that by talking about your problem and about the possible sources of your anxiety, potential solutions and ways of dealing with those anxiety sources begin to crystallise in your mind.

If, for any reason, it is not possible to share your problems with anyone else, just *write* them down as fast as they come up in your mind. This, too, can often both alleviate some of the symptoms and help you find a possible way of dealing with them.

The most effective way of dealing with anxiety symptoms is by doing your *autogenic training* properly, regularly and frequently. Apart from the *standard exercises*, which will be of enormous value in reducing your stress and anxiety, you will derive great benefit from the *anxiety-offloading exercise* as well as from the *anger-offloading* and *screaming exercises*, all described in lesson 5. Don't forget that sometimes the symptoms of anxiety can be due to masked or repressed anger, depression or frustration.

The deep AT state that most of us can achieve after prolonged and frequent use of the standard autogenic training exercises can be used to systematically desensitise people against any phobias they may have, thus enabling them to overcome them. 'My neck and shoulders are heavy', used as a *partial exercise*, is of great benefit in trying to deal with symptoms of severe anxiety, especially of the phobic type, as it can be used anywhere and anytime. Practise it as soon as you feel stress building up to uncomfortable levels, or when you become aware of your phobia taking over.

The *short exercise* is also of considerable help, especially if used frequently during the day when your anxiety symptoms are very severe, in order to top up the general beneficial effects of the full AT exercises. You can also use *positive affirmations*, *guided imagery* and *guided visualisations* in order to combat some of the symptoms of anxiety, though here you must work out for yourself what could be helpful. For instance, if your main source of anxiety is the fact that you have no confidence in yourself, you could include the affirmation, 'I know that I am full of confidence'. (See lesson 9.)

If you suffer from a particular phobia, you can proceed as follows. Get into an AT state, and start very slowly acting out, in your AT state, whatever it is that you are afraid of doing. **It is extremely important to do this slowly and gently.** Take, for instance, fear of going out of the house. First, imagine in your deeply relaxed state that you walk towards the front door. **Cancel immediately if you start getting too anxious.** Be slow, patient and gentle with yourself. Once you can do this without getting anxious, go so far as to open the door. Repeat this in your AT state until, once again, you no longer feel anxious. Next, take one step outside and then come back in. Again, repeat this until there is no anxiety associated with it.

Go on repeating the steps until you have overcome your phobia in your AT state. Once that has been achieved, you can start doing the same thing in real life, using the short exercise, or the partial exercise, repeatedly. Provided that you take it all very slowly and gently over a long period – depending on the extent of your fear – you will find that you are able to overcome almost any phobia. But you must be patient, kind and gentle with yourself. Don't get angry or upset if from time to time you seem to be taking three steps backwards for every two steps forwards. This is part of the whole process, and the important thing to remember is that in the long run you will be able to achieve your goal, whatever it may be.

§16 Arthritis

Unfortunately, there is not enough space in this book to discuss every subdivision of this wide subject, and so I will make only the broadest of comments. More information can be obtained from the many books on the various forms of the disease, or from the relevant organisations (Appendix 2).

Arthritis is of two types, acute and chronic. Of the acute types, the commonest are rheumatoid arthritis, infective arthritis (usually of one joint), polymyalgia rheumatica and gout. The commonest of the chronic varieties are osteo-arthritis and rheumatoid arthritis. Polymyalgia rheumatica is a painful inflammatory condition which usually affects the muscles of the shoulders, chest and arms, although occasionally it may also affect the muscles around the pelvis.

In the acute varieties, as well as the pain, discomfort, swelling and redness which may occur locally in the affected joints and associated muscles, there are more general symptoms such as overall malaise and unwellness, mild fever, headaches, tiredness, loss of appetite, loss of weight, sweating, and general muscle pain, aching and tenderness. In chronic arthritis there are usually very few general symptoms. Chronic pain, and possible deformity and loss of function in the affected joints and their associated muscles and tendons, are the usual ones. It is important to remember that some forms of arthritis, such as rheumatoid, can start as 'acute' and then go into the chronic stage. Sometimes an acute exacerbation can also occur during the chronic phase. Because of the very wide range of conditions classified under the umbrella name 'arthritis', it is very important, if you think you may be suffering from it, to consult your GP so that a proper diagnosis can be made, as the specific treatments depend to a large degree on the underlying causes.

Once a proper diagnosis has been made, apart from the specific treatments that may be offered by the GP and by complementary practitioners, there are things that you can do yourself in order to improve your general condition, with a view to limiting the full impact of the disease.

Weight reduction is very important if you are overweight, as the extra weight will put unnecessary strain on the affected joints, which are probably already feeling delicate. If you are suffering from *acute arthritis*, *resting* the affected parts may be of paramount importance in reducing both the inflammation and the possibility of deformity, whereas in the *chronic phase, movement and physiotherapy* (which can include hydrotherapy) may help in preventing the onset of stiffness and loss of function.

A *nutritious diet* with plenty of fresh fruit and vegetables is also important, and **in some of the more specific types of arthritis certain substances should be avoided:** for example, anyone suffering from gout should avoid alcohol, especially port. In some types of arthritis people often find that, in addition to the supplements discussed in §6, such things as fish liver oils, oil of evening primrose, selenium and zinc can be of great benefit, particularly for reducing pain. Since different conditions call for different remedies, it is best to consult a qualified practitioner about them. Some of the major healthfood shops have qualified dispensers who can advise on such matters.

It may also be worth consulting a qualified *homoeopath or herbalist* (Chinese or Indian), as some of their treatments can be of great benefit even in cases where conventional treatment has been found to be ineffective or to have too many side-effects. *Acupuncture* can also help, especially as far as the reduction of pain and distress is concerned. Other therapies which can be of immense value, especially where muscles are involved, include *massage, reflexology, physiotherapy* and *hydrotherapy*.

Autogenic training can be effective in a number of ways in arthritic conditions. First, by reducing muscle tension around the inflamed joints AT helps to reduce the pain and discomfort, which is often due more to the tension and spasm of the muscles around the affected joints than to the joints themselves. Secondly, it improves the circulation to the affected areas, thereby enabling the natural healing chemicals of the body, as well as any medications, to get working more adequately and effectively. Thirdly, it can be used to reduce the distress associated with the condition, as well as the pain (§42), thus enabling you to deal with chronic arthritis in a much more positive way. Finally, it can help to make you feel that you are taking an active role in your own management and well-being. To empower yourself in this way can only be a good thing.

In cases of rheumatoid arthritis and, possibly, some other forms of inflammatory arthritis, it has been found that chronic repression of the so-called negative emotions, especially sadness and anger, can be significant contributory factors, both in triggering the disease and in perpetuating it. Here, the *offloading exercises*, especially the *screaming*, *crying* and *anger* ones (lesson 5), can be of paramount importance, both as a preventive measure and to reduce the symptoms once the condition has set in. If you become aware of how many repressed, unresolved emotions you are carrying and find that the offloading exercises are inadequate in dealing with them, it may well be worthwhile seeking the help of a qualified *therapist* or *counsellor*.

You can also use *advanced positive affirmations* (lesson 10) to relieve arthritic conditions. Make up your own formula, using warmth, heaviness or coolness, depending on which you feel is right for you, and concentrate on the joint or the area of the muscle that is affected. For instance, you can use the following:

'My shoulder [or other affected joint or area] is warm (heavy, cool).'

You can incorporate this anywhere in the exercise that feels appropriate, including the deepest point of your relaxation. Many other phrases are given elsewhere. Preferably, though, make up your own to suit your specific needs. (See also lesson 9.)

§17 Asthma

Asthma is a condition characterised by restriction of the breathing passages, leading to difficulty in breathing and to wheezing. It can be caused by a number of factors, including allergy to airborne materials such as dust, chemicals and other pollutants, as well as by certain foods. It is important to realise that these allergens vary markedly from one individual to the next, and even in the same individual the effects can be markedly altered from one time to the next by underlying factors such as emotions and stress. There is believed to be a genetic causal factor in some individuals. In others, factors such as lung infections, exercise, stress and emotions, particularly repressed powerful ones such as anger, frustration and depression, can play an important part.

As with any other condition, **the diagnosis of asthma should be confirmed by a qualified practitioner**, just to ensure that there is no other serious underlying condition giving rise to the shortness of breath and wheezing.

What can I do about my asthma?

Once the diagnosis has been made, there are a number of ways, both conventional and complementary, of alleviating the condition and reducing its severity.

If there are specific factors such as infection causing the asthma, these should be treated in the first place. And any allergens known to trigger an attack should also be avoided. *Diet* can be important, particularly as regards avoiding food-stuffs which exacerbate the condition. Selenium has been shown to be useful in reducing the frequency and severity of attacks in a number of individuals. Small amounts of *gentle, rhythmic exercise*, which may include deep breathing, can be helpful, as it increases the air supply to the lungs. Conventional treatment includes inhalers and medications that will reduce the sensitivity of the air passages as well as improve their functioning. These can be used both to prevent an acute attack and as a treatment, once an attack has started. *Physiotherapy* and *massage* can be useful, especially if you have a lot of phlegm and mucus. Other therapies known to be helpful are *homœopathy*, *herbal medicines* and *acupuncture*. *Autogenic training* is also helpful. It reduces any background stress or anxiety, which can be important contributory factors. It alters the body's physiology and chemistry in the direction of healthier functioning. In both these ways it can act as a preventive measure. It can also help in an acute attack by reducing the anxiety and fear specifically associated with the condition, thus enabling the sufferer to breathe more calmly and comfortably, and by so doing reduce the excessive use of inhalers and the like.

The *offloading exercises* (lesson 5), especially those to do with anger, frustration and crying, can be particularly important when you are trying to deal with any repressed or underlying emotions that may be contributing towards an asthmatic attack. And here the help of a *counsellor* or a *psychotherapist* can be invaluable.

I have found that the *standard exercise*, 'It breathes me', can be very useful to those suffering from asthma or difficulty in breathing, for whatever reason, whether psychological or physical. This can include a past history of pneumonia or other lung disease. However, a very few individuals find that they cannot cope with this particular exercise, and have to leave it out of the standard exercises or reduce the number of repetitions (see lesson 6). It's perfectly all right, if this is the case. You will find that doing so will not affect the eventual level of relaxation that you achieve, or the ensuing benefits. Some asthmatics benefit from the use of *positive affirmations*. If this includes you, you may find some of the following phrases useful, in addition to the *standard and partial exercises*. You can, of course, make up your own sentences, which may be more suited to your particular needs (lessons 9 and 10).

'My breathing is calm and regular.'
'My chest is warm (cool, heavy).'
'My throat is warm (cool).'

'My chest (lungs) open(s) out fully, effortlessly and completely.'
'My breathing is calm and comfortable.'
'My breathing is comfortable and effortless.'
'My breathing is smooth and easy.'
'My lungs open out fully and freely with every breath.'
'There is no space in my life for wheezing.'
'I know that I have no time for breathlessness or wheezing.'
'I know that my lungs are healthy.'

§18 Backache and neckache

Backache and neckache are two of the commonest debilitating conditions in the West. They can affect any part of the spine: from the base of the skull right down to the tip of the tail-bone (see figure 8, p. 68). The conditions that can cause backache and neckache are numerous, ranging from the ordinary sprain, fibrositis and lumbago to arthritis, poor posture and inflammatory, infective and malignant conditions – although, fortunately, this last is NOT one of the commoner causes. Backache and neckache can also be caused by stress and repressed emotions. In fact this is not an unusual source of the trouble, especially in those whose condition does not seem to respond to the usual treatments. Even when there is another, primary, cause, stress and the repression of powerful emotions can certainly aggravate and exacerbate the pain, discomfort and distress of the condition.

If you have a backache which seems to persist and there is no obvious cause for it, such as lifting a heavy object awkwardly, **do consult your doctor so that he can try to find the cause**. The treatment depends on the cause, so I will just make a few broad comments about what treatments are generally available. Do choose your therapy carefully, and be guided by those who are looking after you. The management of the condition also varies according to whether the problem is acute or chronic.

What can I do?

In an acute back or neck condition, it is usually advisable to *rest the part*, in order to allow it to heal more quickly. Rest may entail the use of a collar or a spinal corset, depending on the severity of the condition or the symptoms associated with it. Once the acute phase has eased, then controlled movement and mobilisation can be of benefit.

Heat, via hot water bottles, infra-red lamp or heated pads, or some of the proprietary liniments and creams, is usually quite helpful. *Pain-killers* may be necessary, as may *other conventional medications* designed to reduce the inflammation or remedy some other underlying condition. *Homoeopathic and herbal remedies*, as well as *acupuncture, osteopathy, physiotherapy, hydrotherapy, chiropractic, massage* and *spiritual healing*, can be helpful, depending to some extent on the underlying cause of the trouble.

One of the commonest causes of chronic backache and neckache is **poor posture**, which is due to the way you stand, sit, walk or sleep. Most people think that backache at night and in the morning is caused by too soft a bed, and although this might be the case, especially if the bed has seen many years of stalwart service and consequently sags in the middle, what they seem to forget is that they can get backache if their bed is **too hard**. I have come across many cases in which backache has got worse after the bed has been replaced by a hard 'orthopaedic' one, just because the salesman in the shop or, more commonly, the advertisement in the Press happened to be very persuasive! THE MOST IMPORTANT THING IS THAT YOUR BED MUST BE RIGHT AND COMFORTABLE FOR YOU. It is a good idea to try numerous beds, until you find the one that suits you and your particular shape or build.

Mobility can be very important for *chronic backache and neckache* – assuming that there is no serious underlying cause – because it can prevent the affected parts from becoming fixed or deformed. So *physiotherapy, hydrotherapy, massage, aromatherapy, osteopathy* as well as *chiropractic* can all have important roles to play in the management of chronic pain and stiffness. I have found that spiritual healing seems to be a particularly effective treatment in the relief of symptoms, especially in my hands. *Losing weight* is important, if you happen to be overweight and suffering from backache, as in that way you can reduce the physical strains on your back and on the rest of your musculoskeletal system.

Antogenic training helps by reducing the tension in those large muscles of the back and neck (see lesson 2); as they relax and the spasm diminishes, so does the pain. A great deal of backache and neckache is due to the tension in the muscles surrounding the affected parts. As a lot of pain can also be due to repressed and unresolved emotions, the *offloading exercises* (lesson 5) can be of tremendous value. You may have to use the full range, until you discover the ones that are particularly helpful to you. This is because the underlying emotions causing the problem may not be immediately apparent, especially if you have been repressing them into the area of your back or neck for a long time, and have been totally unaware of doing it. Remember that the possible underlying emotion(s) will vary from one time to the next, and you may have to vary the exercises according to your changing circumstances and the associated emotions and feelings.

Another way of utilising your AT to help you deal with the symptoms is to use a specific *affirmation* as a part of your standard exercises, such as 'My back is warm (heavy [or both])', or 'My neck and shoulders are heavy and warm', and concentrate at the same time on the painful area(s). It may help if you try to imagine, for instance, a hand or other source of warmth massaging the affected part of your neck or back. (See also lesson 9).

§19 Blood pressure problems

High blood pressure, or hypertension, is a very common condition, the incidence of which increases with age. Although in a few instances there may be a treatable underlying cause, most of those who suffer from it seem to develop it for no apparent reason. It can be totally asymptomatic. The condition is often discovered quite by chance, when one's blood pressure is being taken for some other reason. It is also discovered when a person suffers one of its side-effects, such as a stroke or heart attack. Occasionally, high blood pressure may cause a few symptoms, including aching in the back of the head or on top of the neck, which often occurs in the early hours of the morning, palpitations, breathlessness, nose-bleeds, chest pains, dizziness, pains in the legs on exertion, and visual disturbances.

It is best to **see your doctor if you have any of the above symptoms**, or even if you just think that you have raised blood pressure, in order to confirm the diagnosis or to have it ruled out. Beyond the age of thirty-five, it is always advisable to have your blood pressure checked at least once every five years, so that if you do start suffering from it, it can be detected early, before complications such as kidney disease, visual problems, heart failure, strokes and heart attacks develop.

What can I do?

Once you have been diagnosed as suffering from raised blood pressure, there is a lot you can do to improve the situation. By far the best way of going about it is to choose a natural way, as most conventional treatments have some sort of side-effects. *Homœopathic* and *herbal* remedies may be quite helpful from this point of view.

Lose weight if you are overweight. Cut down on or, if you

can, *stop drinking coffee and strong teas. Give up smoking and avoid places where other people are smoking. Reduce your fluid, including alcohol, and your salt and fat intake. Increase your supplement intake, especially vitamins C, E and fibre. Avoid animal fats, and use vegetable oils for cooking and margarine instead of butter.*

The *standard autogenic training exercises* can help, by reducing stress and cholesterol levels as well as increasing the circulation to the limbs which is one of the ways of reducing blood pressure. And the *offloading exercises*, especially those dealing with anger and frustration, can play an important role in the management of hypertension. Remember that although raised blood pressure sometimes settles down permanently, the trainee usually has to keep on practising the exercises for an indefinite period in order to keep his blood pressure in check.

Positive affirmations (lesson 9) can also be used to reduce blood pressure, by opening the peripheral circulation with a sentence such as:

'My arms and legs are warm.'

If these measures do not help, or your blood pressure is too high, then your GP will obviously give you conventional medical treatments which can be used in conjunction with the measures discussed above.

§20 Blushing

This condition, which can be very distressing to the sufferer, seems to be greatly alleviated by the use of *autogenic training*. It not only helps to reduce blushing itself, but also helps the sufferer to overcome the fear of blushing, which in itself may often aggravate the condition. The problem can be further alleviated by the use of *positive affirmations*, such as:

'My neck and shoulders are heavy and warm.'
'My feet are warm.'

In addition to being a regular part of the AT exercise, one of these sentences can be used as soon as a situation arises that may cause blushing, as can the *partial exercise*, 'My neck and shoulders are heavy' (lesson 2).

§21 Cancer

Cancer is a very emotive and scary word, and until quite recently most people avoided mentioning it, tending to skirt around the subject instead. However, unless and until we are truly open about it, neither the sufferers nor those who are looking after and supporting them can draw upon the body's tremendous reserves in order to help fend off the disease.

Cancer is caused by the fast and irregular growth of abnormal cells, which have the capacity not only of invading the normal tissues surrounding them but also, in certain situations, of spreading to other tissues and organs well beyond the primary site. This is not a single disease, as almost every known cell in the body can go cancerous, and thus every tissue and organ can be affected.

The process of cell division in the body is constantly going on, and as a result numerous new cells are being produced. For instance, the whole lining of the gut (from mouth to anus) is replaced every thirty-six hours. This constant production of new cells is necessary for the proper functioning, repair and replacement of worn-out and diseased cells. A tiny proportion of these new cells, in a perfectly healthy person, is either abnormal or cancerous. Most of the time these cells are destroyed and mopped up by the body's natural defences, and cause no problems. But sometimes, and for a variety of reasons, destruction of the abnormal cells does not occur, and this leads to the start of the condition that we call 'cancer'. Currently **a quarter of all UK deaths are caused by this condition**.

What are the factors that make us more susceptible to cancer?

Age is an important factor, as by and large the incidence of cancer increases with age. Certain cancers, though, have a predilection for specific ages: for instance, some bone cancers and acute leukaemia particularly affect children; testicular cancer in men and cervical cancer in women both occur in early middle age. Other contributory factors are *smoking* (causing lung and stomach cancers), *alcohol* (stomach and liver cancers), *excessive sun* (certain skin cancers), and *exposure to chemical irritants* such as chromium, aniline dyes, asbestos and coal dust, to name but a few.

Stress plays a very important role, not only in the inception of the disease but also in its spread and progress. (See §1.) The adverse effects of both acute and chronic stress on the immune system was mentioned earlier: it is essential that we have an intact and perfectly functioning *immune system* so that it can seek out and destroy the cancer cells that are constantly being produced in our bodies. So to help to improve our immune system, we must learn to control and deal with our stress problems. Another factor that has been shown to interfere with the proper functioning of the immune system, making us more susceptible to the effects of cancer production, is the *repression of the so-called negative emotions* such as frustration, anger and sadness. (See lesson 5.)

Other factors that may also play a part are *inadequate diet and nutritional supplements*, and the individual's *personality*. Cancer-prone people tend to be the sort who are constantly doing things – at work, at home, for others. If they are not always on the go, or if they decide to give some time to themselves, they tend to feel guilty. They generally tend to be the 'workaholics', the perfectionists and the go-getters. They often have great difficulty in saying 'No' to others, and in asking others for help.

Since cancer can affect every tissue and organ in the body, the symptoms are extremely varied, depending on which organs or tissues are affected. But there are a few non-specific symptoms that should alert us to the possibility of the existence of cancer in the system. **Do remember, though, that each of these symptoms can occur in numerous other conditions as well. So don't panic or convince yourself that you have cancer, if you do have one of the symptoms. Just consult your doctor, for a proper diagnosis.** The symptoms include: fatigue and lethargy; unexplained weight loss, particularly if large and sudden; unusual persistent pain; inexplicable headache; change in bowel habit and loss of appetite; persistent cough or hoarse voice. **And if you find a lump or swelling anywhere in or on your body, no matter how insignificant or painless, it is well worthwhile consulting your doctor** so that he or she can make a proper diagnosis.

How can I help myself?

The most important aspect of cancer therapy is **prevention**, and it is worth repeating here what I said at the beginning of this section. Avoid the sort of pollutants, activities, and so on that are known to cause cancer. Avoid smoking. Drink alcohol only in moderation. Deal with your personality, with stress and with your repressed emotions. If you are unfortunate enough to get cancer, YOU MUST BE CLEAR ABOUT THE DIAGNOSIS – because if you are not, you will be unable to utilise your own immense healing powers and direct them towards the source of your illness.

Diet and nutritional supplements (see §6) *are extremely important. Homœopathy and herbal medicine can also play an important role, as can therapy such as counselling, psychotherapy and spiritual healing, especially in controlling the symptoms. Your GP or hospital consultant will institute any conventional treatment that may be required.*

Autogenic training can work very effectively in enabling you to reduce your stress level, not the least cause of which may be your own cancer. AT can also help you to develop a positive mental attitude towards yourself, your cancer and your health and well-being, which will be of the utmost importance; and the *offloading exercises* (lesson 5) help you to deal with your repressed and unworked-through feelings such as anger and depression. Another way of deriving maximum benefit from the AT state is to use it for *positive affirmations*, and *guided visualisations* and *imagery* (lessons 9, 10 and 11).

§22   Cholesterol and lipids

These substances, which are constituents of *fats*, are essential
for certain body functions. However, excess of certain lipids,
as well as of cholesterol, can lead to a number of serious
conditions. First and foremost, it can lead to the furring-up of
the body's blood vessels (arteries, mainly), a condition commonly known as atherosclerosis. It can lead to high blood
pressure, heart attacks, strokes and poor circulation in the
legs – causing difficulty in walking – and, in extreme cases,
gangrene (especially in combination with smoking).

What can I do?

The most important thing to do in order to reduce the
incidence of the conditions just mentioned is to **prevent them
from happening**. This can be achieved by cutting down your
intake of fats, especially saturated and animal fats, to an
absolute minimum: so *dietary restriction* is all-important.
Avoid fat on meat, and reduce your intake of red meats to the
minimum, as even the leanest of the red meats may have as
much as 15 per cent of fat. You can further improve the
situation by *replacing your intake of saturated animal fats with
polyunsaturated fats*, such as those present in corn oil and
sunflower oil. Olive oil, rich in monounsaturated fats, is also
good. For butter substitute vegetable equivalents. Other
foods that help to reduce blood cholesterol and fats include
aubergines, garlic, onions, walnut, pecan nut, peas and
beans, rye, oats, barley and soya beans, and many foods with
high fibre and low fat content. Fresh fruits and vegetables,
especially the green varieties such as lettuce, cabbage,
broccoli, watercress and spinach, are also helpful. Other
useful supplements which have been reported to help
reduce cholesterol and lipids are high dose magnesium,
vitamin C, zinc, selenium, nicotinic acid, calcium, Omega 3
and 6 fatty acids (in fish oils, green vegetables, walnuts,

pecan nuts and linseed oil capsules) and lecithin (phosphodyl choline) at a minimum dose of 1 gramme two or three times a day.

REMEMBER THAT, DESPITE ALL THE DIETARY RESTRICTIONS THAT YOU MAY IMPOSE UPON YOURSELF, IT IS NOT POSSIBLE TO REDUCE BLOOD CHOLESTEROL BELOW A CERTAIN LEVEL, since up to 75 per cent of it is manufactured in the liver, primarily under the influence of the chemical adrenalin and noradrenalin, which are released when you are under stress. Consequently, one of the most effective ways of reducing the blood cholesterol level is to practise *autogenic training*. It has been shown conclusively that by reducing background stress with the *standard exercises*, blood cholesterol normalises, even in those individuals whom nothing else seems to have greatly helped.

Exercise has also been shown to reduce blood cholesterol effectively, especially in conjunction with AT.

It follows that, in order to try to reduce the levels of lipids and cholesterol in the blood, the best plan of action is to combine an effective diet with exercise and stress management through autogenic training.

§23 Circulation problems

A great many people suffer from cold hands and feet, and there are specific medical conditions that can cause or aggravate the situation. So if this is your problem, it is advisable to go and see your doctor, to ensure that there is no serious underlying reason for your poor circulation.

What can I do?

The general advice on how to improve your circulation is very similar to that already given in the sections on angina and blood pressure (14 and 19). However, there is **one crucial factor** contributing towards or aggravating poor circulation – even, in extreme cases, leading to gangrene – and that is **smoking. So if you suffer from poor circulation, it is imperative that you stop smoking.**

Diet is very important (see §§14 and 19 again), and there are also some specific supplements that help to improve circulation. These include vitamin C and the B group of vitamins, particularly nicotinic acid.

The *standard autogenic training exercises*, especially the warmth ones, are extremely beneficial for this condition, even when there are underlying physical problems. Some individuals, prescribed vasodilator drugs – designed to improve the peripheral circulation – by their GP, have managed either to come off them altogether or to reduce their intake substantially. The warmth and the improved circulation effected by the standard exercises can be considerably enhanced by the use of specific *positive affirmations*, such as:

'My ears (nose, fingers, toes, calves [and so on]) are warm.'
'The circulation to my —— [affected part] is free and easy.'
'I feel a glow of warmth in my —— .'
'It circulates freely.'

'My circulation is free and unimpeded.'
'My blood circulates freely and easily in all my organs (parts, tissues [and so on]).'
'Warmth improves my circulation.'
'Warmth improves circulation to my ——— .'
'Warmth heals my circulation.'
'Warmth heals my ——— .'

You can, of course, make up your own phrases to suit your personality or situation. (See also lesson 9.)

§24 Colitis

This is a condition that affects the large bowel (intestine), and is characterised by abdominal pain, which may be achy and continuous or sharp and colicky. It can also be associated with diarrhoea, frequency of motions or constipation. There may be bleeding and the passing of mucus, depending on the severity of the condition. There may also be a constant feeling of wanting to open one's bowels, although the symptom is not greatly relieved by doing so. It can present as an acute condition which sometimes settles down quickly; in other instances, the acute phase can then lead on to a chronic phase. The cause of colitis is not really known, although there are a number of contributory factors such as infection, food allergies such as milk intolerance, and a disturbed immune system. The most important contributory factor seems to be stress and the repression of strong emotions, especially sadness and anger.

If you suffer from any of the above symptoms and they last more than a few days, you **must** consult your GP to try to find out what the underlying problem may be. Once you have a proper diagnosis, then you can proceed with the advice below.

What can I do?

First of all, make sure that you *have plenty of rest* in the *acute phase* of the disease, and that you *have a simple but nutritious diet with plenty of supplements*, especially vitamin C and iron, as the condition can be associated with some degree of anaemia. Avoid smoking. Reduce the fibre in your diet (unless constipation is a problem). If you suspect that you may have an allergy (or allergies), get yourself properly investigated by a qualified nutritionist. If you are found to be allergic to any specific substances, ensure that you avoid them completely. The bowel symptoms can be alleviated by medicines bought across the counter, or prescribed by your doctor or by a homœopath or herbalist. All three can offer beneficial treatments for both the acute and the chronic phases.

During the *chronic phase*, *increase your intake of food*, unless you find that by doing so you aggravate the situation. *Dietary supplements* are as necessary in this phase as in the acute phase.

As stress seems to play a significant role in causing colitis as well as in perpetuating it, it follows that *autogenic training* can have beneficial effects on a number of levels. First, it helps to reduce basic stress, as well as enabling the sufferer to deal more adequately and effectively with whatever stresses he may be subjected to. It helps to maintain the equilibrium of the autonomic nervous system (see §1), and thus to reduce bowel spasms. This in turn helps to reduce the pain, as well as the diarrhoea or constipation. As the movements of the bowel normalise and settle down, so will the inflammation, the bleeding and the passage of mucus, as well as other symptoms such as feeling bloated. The improvement of the trainee's general condition as well as of his immune system, which will necessarily follow, will be of great benefit in helping him to overcome his illness.

Free use of the *offloading exercises* (lesson 5) as well as of the *positive affirmations* (lessons 9 and 10) can be particularly helpful as far as the overall effectiveness of the AT and the relief of the condition are concerned. The positive affirmations can be used both to control symptoms such as pain and diarrhoea or constipation, and to further alleviate the condition itself. Here are just a few of the many phrases that can be used:

'My abdomen [lower or upper, depending on the site of the pain] is warm (heavy, cool).'
'My bowel is comfortable and relaxed.'
'I know that I am healing my bowel.'
'My stomach (bowel) is comfortable, relaxed and pain-free.'
'My bowel action is slow and infrequent.' (For diarrhoea.)
'I am happy with the functioning of my bowel.'

See also §§26, 35 and 61.

§25 Concentration

Many factors can disturb our concentration. There are a number of physical conditions, especially some affecting the nervous system, which can do so. But perhaps the commonest causes of disturbance or reduction in concentration level are simply a lack of determination to pay attention to the subject being discussed and the presence of some degree of stress, anxiety, depression or other underlying psychological problem. When you are learning autogenic training, your concentration during the exercises may at first be poor. (In Part 2 we discussed the reasons for this.) As you progress with the exercises, your ability to concentrate will improve as your ability to relax improves.

If you find that your concentration has deteriorated, especially recently, try to work out why. If you feel that it may be due to some underlying physical condition, do consult your doctor in order to clarify the situation. If there is no underlying problem, you must make a conscious effort to improve your concentration by *paying particular attention to everything*. This may initially be quite hard work. But once you have got into the habit of paying attention, it will become a lot easier.

Make sure that you have an *adequate diet* and plenty of *supplements*, as the vitamin B group is known to help the proper functioning of the nervous system.

Autogenic training is, of course, of great benefit, if your lack of concentration is due to stress, repressed emotions, anxiety or depression. The *standard exercises* will help to reduce background stress, and, as I have said, with that will come a considerable improvement in your concentration, in your everyday life as well as during your AT. The *offloading exercises* can be of immense value in enabling you to deal with any underlying, unresolved emotional problems, as well as anxiety, depression and frustration (lesson 5 and §§15 and 27).

You can, of course, use *positive affirmations* as described in lessons 9 and 10, and in §40. And you could add these:

'I'll pay more attention.'
'I'll remember if I try.'
'I know that I have an excellent memory.'
'I'll concentrate all the time.'
'Concentration is easy, and happens naturally.'

See also §29, on education.

§26 Constipation

This common complaint can be a constant source of distress and annoyance to the sufferer. It can have numerous causes, so if you suffer from it, especially if you have developed the condition recently and without any previous history, consult your doctor. Once a diagnosis has been made, you can use other measures, including AT, to alleviate the condition.

What can I do?

ONE OF THE COMMONEST CAUSES OF CONSTIPATION IS INADEQUATE ROUGHAGE, OR FIBRE, in the diet, AS WELL AS NOT DRINKING ENOUGH, particularly in hot weather. So one of the first things to do is to *increase your consumption of fibre* by eating more fresh fruit, vegetables, wholemeal bread, cereals, and so on, and to *make sure that you are drinking enough.* Fresh fruit juice, including extracts of the whole fruit, and especially prune and fig juice, are particularly helpful. Homœopathic and herbal remedies can also be of use, as can vegetable-based and other kinds of proprietary medicine. However, these should not be taken over long periods, as they can make the bowel even more lazy, and dependent on their regular use.

The use of the *standard AT exercises* usually seems to effectively regulate bowel function within four to eight weeks. It has been found that not only does most trainees' constipation disappear, but also the many symptoms commonly attributed to it, such as feelings of fullness, abdominal discomfort, headache, indigestion and belching, are alleviated. Better sleep, increased appetite and a better body weight have also been reported. These changes, and the alleviation and even total disappearance of constipation, are probably due to the automatic normalisation of the autonomic nervous system (§1). It is interesting to note that in a number of cases constipation did not recur until up to two years after the regular AT exercises had been discontinued.

Apart from regular use of the standard exercises, *positive affirmations* (lessons 9 and 10) can help to alleviate persistent and chronic cases of constipation. Try such phrases as:

'My lower abdomen is warm.'
'My bowels empty regularly and effortlessly.'
'My bowels empty regularly after breakfast (lunch [and so on]).'
'My bowels are automatic and work without laxatives.'
'I don't need laxatives to empty my bowels.'
'It empties regularly and automatically.'

These are just a few examples. The best thing is to formulate your own, as described in lesson 9.

§27 Depression

This is such a common condition that I do not think there is
anyone who is exempt from feeling it from time to time. It
includes feeling sad and just generally low. The problem is
to know at what point ordinary sadness, caused by some
difficult or tragic circumstance, becomes severe enough to be
considered an illness.

Like most other emotional symptoms, its seriousness depends to a large extent on one's perception of one's circumstances. What to one person seems tragic enough to send him
or her into the depths of depression, may make the next
person just sad and upset for a few days, after which he or she
quickly recovers. Depression can present not only as a feeling
of sadness. There are other symptoms, which include tiredness, lethargy, loss of interest in life, apathy; just feeling
awful, especially in the mornings, and for no apparent reason;
lack of energy; decrease in activity and a general slowing
down; feelings of 'Can't be bothered with anything'; loss of
sexual drive; sleep disturbances, especially early-morning
waking; constipation; abnormal variations in weight, both
gaining and losing; disturbance of menstrual periods;
headaches, especially feelings of heaviness or pressure in the
head; self-deprecation, ideas of guilt and shame; excessive
involvement and interest in one's own symptoms, which take
on very large proportions; general malaise and achiness;
and in extremely severe cases, delusions, paranoia and
hallucinations.

It is true that most of us feel one or more of these symptoms
from time to time, depending on our circumstances. It is only
when there is a combination of symptoms, and the feelings
associated with them are excessive or inappropriate, that the
condition becomes an illness rather than a normal reaction of
sadness or grief to some difficult or tragic situation. It is worth
bearing in mind that depression may be associated with or

even result from other emotional problems such as chronic anxiety, frustration or repressed anger, especially directed at oneself. For a great many people, especially women, it is much more socially acceptable to be depressed and tearful than to feel, let alone exhibit, annoyance, anger or rage.

How can I help myself?

THE MOST IMPORTANT THING IS TO ACKNOWLEDGE THAT YOU MAY BE DEPRESSED, AND TO GIVE YOURSELF PERMISSION TO EXPERI-ENCE FEELINGS OF SADNESS AND DEPRESSION. If you do this, you can often make life somewhat easier for yourself, and your feelings more tolerable. It's a bit like letting off steam, which leaves you feeling that there is less of it left to continue causing trouble and needing to be dealt with. Once you have acknowledged that you are depressed, stressed and dis-tressed, sit down and carefully list the circumstances or situations that are making you upset now, or have done so in the past (lesson 5). Having done that, you will be in a much better position to do something about it – either to try to change the situation or, if that is not possible, as in the case of bereavement, to offload the feelings by *talking about them with a close and understanding friend or relation, or, better still, with a trained counsellor or therapist.*

Improve your general health by following a *good diet* with the necessary *supplements*, especially if loss of appetite is one of your problems. Increase your intake of fibre, if consti-pation is another symptom, by eating plenty of wholegrain cereals and bread, fruit and vegetables. St John's wort, a herbal remedy which is available from most reputable health food stores, can be very effective in relieving the symptoms of depression.

Autogenic training will, of course, help with the underlying stress and anxiety. One of the best ways of getting rid of feelings of sadness, distress or depression is to do freely the *offloading exercises* described in lesson 5, particularly those associated with anger, crying and frustration. Some depressed people find that at first they get more out of these exercises than out of the standard AT exercises. If this applies to you, it is perfectly all right to try to empty out your grief and anger first, in order to get the maximum benefit from your *standard exercises* later. Other people suffering from depression may be totally unaware of the amount of sadness and tears that they are carrying, and only get in touch with them while doing their AT. This does not mean that AT is not good or beneficial for them. On the contrary, AT is usually a very important step in their long search for true self-improvement and empowerment. For once they acknowledge these feelings and give themselves permission to offload them, they will make contact with their deep inner peace and contentment, and the repressed feelings will no longer be there to accumulate and cause trouble in the future.

Positive affirmations can also be of considerable help in alleviating other symptoms that may be associated with depression (see lessons 9 and 10), as well as the sections on specific medical conditions in Part 3.

If, after following the advice given above, you find that there is no improvement, or if you start feeling worse, it is best for you to consult your doctor for further advice and help.

§28   Dieting

Most people associate the word 'diet' with trying to lose weight. However, it is important to remember that specific dieting can be a central part of both preventive medicine – such as a low animal fat diet in order to help prevent coronary heart disease – and curative medicine. Proper diet is an extremely important factor in the management of diabetes, with or without medication. Dieting can also be very useful as an adjunct to the holistic approach to the improvement of health, and in fighting diseases such as AIDS and cancer.

A discussion of the many diets that can be followed is outside the scope of this book, and anyway there are numerous books dealing with them individually. If you have any special needs, consult a dietitian or a nutritionist who specialises in the field. It is important to remember that some people over-eat and put on too much weight as a compensation for psychological problems or repressed emotions and the need for security. If you suspect that you have any such problems, *do consult a counsellor or therapist.* And before embarking on a weight-losing diet, **make sure that there are no underlying physical reasons for your being overweight.**

What can I do?

My main aim here is to indicate how *autogenic training* can enable you to stick to any particular diet that you have chosen or that has been prescribed for you. AT can help to relieve any background stress or anxiety. If there are associated emotional problems, the *offloading exercises* (lesson 5) can be an extremely useful tool in dealing with them and thus making dieting easier. But the most important aspect of AT in this context is the use of *positive affirmations* or *visualisations* of one sort or another, in order to help you to stick to your diet (lesson 9). Be mindful of how you make up your formulae, as they must reflect what you hope to achieve.

If you want to use a particular diet in order to lose weight, you have to work out what aspect is the most difficult for you. For instance, do you eat too much at each meal? Do you eat in between meals? Do you eat too many meals? Or do you eat too many sweet and fattening things? Once you realise where your main problem lies, you can use a specific type of affirmation to control it. If you have more than one problem, you may have to use more than one affirmation. For examples of the kind of affirmations that may be useful, see §41 on obesity. The following phrases are examples for someone who has difficulty in sticking to a particular diet:

'I know that I will stick to my diet.'
'I find my —— (diabetic, non-lipid [and so on]) diet pleasant and enjoyable.'
'I enjoy my diet.'
'It is easy to stick to my diet.'

§29 Education

Autogenic training can be used successfully as a learning aid by children of primary school age, by adolescents and by young adults. Most of the knowledge available in the field has been obtained by studying students, mainly in Canada and Japan.

AT AND YOUNG CHILDREN

It has not always been thought advisable to teach AT to children younger than eight or nine, as it was found in the late 1950s that below that age they find it difficult both to assimilate the knowledge and to apply it. However, these days a lot of children are more mature than their age would suggest, so children younger than this can probably be taught the technique. All the same, the exercises should be modified. This means, in effect, that *only the heaviness and warmth exercises* (lessons 1, 2 and 3) *and the cooling exercise* (lesson 8) *should be used* for this age group as most children seem to have great difficulty with the concepts of the others, especially the *abdominal warmth exercise* (lesson 7).

The *offloading exercises* (lesson 5) can also be quite useful, especially for those children who have any sort of behavioural problem, whether related to school or to home. In extensive studies of the use of autogenic training in some schools in Canada, with children aged between eight and ten years, a number of beneficial effects were observed by all parties involved – that is, the children, the parents and the teachers. These included:

1 Improvement in eating and sleeping patterns.
2 Reduction in the level of irritability, moodiness and crying.
3 Reduction in hostile and unsociable behaviour.

4   Improvement in relationships with each other as well as with adults.
5   More active participation in play and other group activities, as well as in classwork.
6   Improvement in the quality of homework, as well as better marks.
7   Improvement in paying attention, and in concentration.
8   Improvement in behaviour both at home and at school.
9   Improvement in exam results.

It was found that improvements in the general health of the children also occurred. These included a reduction in the number of complaints of stomach ache and headache; an improvement in the condition of those children who were stuttering, had nervous tics, or were wetting themselves; and a reduction in asthma attacks in the asthmatic children. As the children in the surveys took very easily to AT and generally found it fun to do, not least because of the tremendous improvement it made to their general well-being, I thoroughly recommend it in this modified form as a technique that children can learn and use as a preventive measure, and especially as an investment for the future.

AT AND ADOLESCENTS

There are a number of factors that can interfere with the scholastic achievement of adolescent students, who are going through a great many physiological and psychological changes. These changes include increasing pressure, both at home and at school, for greater achievement, particularly in examinations; the constantly changing demands of their roles in the family and at school; the need to adapt socially, and an awareness of their newly found sexuality, with all the emotional and psychological problems that this can bring; and environmental ones, such as changing schools or moving house.

It was found that when the teenagers in the surveys practised AT regularly, they managed to progress from one phase of their development to another (from pre-, through mid- to post-teens) with far fewer problems than might have been expected. Other benefits that were observed were:

1　Improvement in concentration and in their ability to learn, especially in the AT state and with the use of *positive affirmations*.
2　Improvement in self-discipline and in the standard of homework.
3　Ability to study for much longer periods.
4　Reduction in extraneous emotional problems interfering with studies.
5　Improved sleep patterns.
6　Improved ability to cope generally.
7　Reduction in anxiety, including that associated with examinations.
8　Better and friendlier relationships with other students, parents and teachers.
9　Increased flexibility in fitting in with both home and school arrangements.
10　Reduction in psychosomatic symptoms such as headaches, stomach aches and nervous tics.
11　Improved ability to achieve. Even the so-called under-achievers were found to perform much better and to gain much better marks than expected, compared with past performance.

AT AND YOUNG ADULTS

The results obtained in large groups of college students confirmed for this older age group the benefits that were achieved by the adolescents. Additionally, it was found that a great many of the students who had not originally been expected to get into technical colleges or university managed to do so, as their performance had improved so much. Other benefits were:

1　Improved stability of personality.
2　Improvement in intelligence of up to 20 per cent according to IQ tests. This was probably because, being more relaxed and composed, the students were able to utilise their intelligence more effectively.
3　Marked improvement in concentration, not only in its quality but also in duration, which almost tripled in the large groups studied.

4   Marked increase in the length of study periods, as the students were able to repeatedly refresh themselves while they were studying, using both the short and standard exercises (lesson 1), thereby increasing their stamina.

See the suggestions for *positive affirmations*, and other ways of increasing students' ability to learn, on pages 126 and 132. This procedure is equally effective with the older age groups.

Autogenic training has also been taught to teachers, accountants, military cadets, doctors and nurses with a view to improving their learning skills, with equally beneficial results.

All that these descriptions demonstrate is that AT IS AN EXTREMELY USEFUL EDUCATIONAL TOOL, even for children as young as eight. All the benefits described had been achieved merely with the *standard exercises*, which permit the mind to carry on with its own self-improvement processes. The effects can be further enhanced, as already mentioned, by the use of the *positive affirmations* (lesson 9). See also §25, on concentration.

What can I do?

Positive affirmations can be quite effective in dealing with young people's problems, both physical and emotional. It is best to work out for yourself, with the help of parents or teachers if necessary, where your possible problems and shortcomings lie, so that the affirmations can concentrate on those specific areas. Here are a few examples (see also lessons 9 and 10):

'I know that I am confident.'
'I am calm and creative.'
'Homework is easy and fun.'
'School is fun and enjoyable.'
'I like and enjoy my school.'
'I love doing my homework.'
'I like my teachers.'
'I love my parents (mother, father, sisters, brothers).'
'I enjoy going to school.'
'I enjoy playing sports.'

Another very good way of increasing your ability to learn and of boosting your scholastic achievements is to use *guided visualisations* or *imagery* in an AT state. This can be done in two ways. *Either* you can get into an AT state and then rehearse or revise whatever it is that you want to learn or memorise. This will considerably improve the ease and speed of your learning. *Or*, if you have difficulties in understanding a particular subject, you can think of that subject and then get into an AT state. The answer to the problem may come to you when you reach a deep AT state. This may not happen the very first time, so be patient and do not expect it to happen automatically. When the mind is ready, it will allow the answer to come through. (See also lessons 10 and 11.)

§30 Flying

Before discussing the beneficial effects of autogenic training in aviation or flying, it is important that I point out the problems encountered both by the occasional long-distance traveller and by air crews, on whom the effects are much more prolonged and profound. These effects are associated either with the prospective traveller's fear of flying, or with the physiological changes which result from flying and which are generally known as 'jet lag'.

'Jet lag' is now an established expression, and all long-distance travellers experience it. It is rather a misnomer, though, as travellers experienced it even when they were flying in non-jet aircraft. It is a syndrome that consists of a number of symptoms, all or some of which may be present in any individual traveller, to a greater or lesser degree. They include *tiredness, fatigue, lassitude, anxiety, irritability, depression; and disturbance of motivation, performance, mood and sleep.* There may also be a *reduction in powers of decision-making and logical thought,* as well as *some degree of short-term memory loss.* These last are, of course, of the utmost significance to those who need to be able to make rapid decisions and accurate judgements.

So although the problems associated with jet lag are just a nuisance to the ordinary holidaymaker, who can afford the time to adapt to 'jet lag' symptoms, they are extremely serious to the flight crew and the businessman, who have no extra time to overcome such problems during their working routine. Apart from the main cause of jet lag, which is the body's inability to adjust to the rapid changes of time zone necessitated by high-speed long-distance air travel, a number of other factors contribute to it, including alterations in diet, humidity, noise levels, hydration levels of the traveller and cabin pressurisation; alterations in sleep patterns; and the consumption of a variety of drugs including tranquillisers, sleeping tablets, alcohol and caffeine (in coffee and tea). Fatigue and tiredness, two of the commonest jet lag symptoms, may be associated with a number of pre-flight factors, such as inadequate rest, excessive or unaccustomed exercise (swimming, skiing, for instance), the stress of getting to the airport, flight delays, passport and customs formalities.

The normal, comfortable air humidity for most people in their living-rooms is 40–60 per cent. During a long flight it can drop to as low as 3 per cent, which can give rise to dryness in the respiratory tract and fatigue, as well as an increased risk of infection through the respiratory tract such as colds, sore throat and bronchitis. It can also cause dryness of the skin, although general dehydration is uncommon provided that enough non-alcoholic fluids are consumed during the flight. **Coffee and alcohol**, which act as diuretics, **should be avoided** as, together with the low humidity in the aircraft, they can lead to dehydration. A diuretic is a substance that removes fluid from the body and pushes it out through the kidneys. Your degree of thirst during a flight is not a good indication of the level of hydration or of your fluid requirement. You should drink as much fluid as you feel is necessary, irrespective of whether or not you are thirsty. One other possible side-effect of low humidity is increased static electricity when you touch metal objects.

The detrimental effects of noise can be both physiological and psychological. The physiological aspect mainly applies to the air crew, who in the long term may suffer some deterioration of their hearing. The psychological aspect is more important in the short term, as it can lead to increased difficulties in communication and hence increased irritability, stress and fatigue in both staff and passengers.

However, the most important factor contributing to tiredness on a long-haul journey is the disturbance of the body's natural twenty-four-hour rhythm: the so-called *circadian rhythm*. It is important to realise that most of the systems of the body work in a regular cycle of roughly twenty-four hours' duration. There are exceptions to this, of course, such as the menstrual cycle in women. These rhythms are controlled by the brain, but the bašic twenty-four-hour cycle is maintained by a number of factors, of which the most important are light and dark. Other significant factors are meal-times, and other physical and social activities. The many hormones and other chemicals which are responsible for the proper functioning of all the cycles are not only interdependent, but are also dependent on the proper functioning of the nervous system and the brain. The release of the hormones and chemicals, and their relation to each other, can become disturbed if there are any changes of the kind that affect the brain and the nervous system, such as broken sleep.

In addition to the rhythmical changes caused by hormones and chemicals, it has been found that the body's temperature and the brain's intellectual and task-performance functions also alter rhythmically, with the lowest temperature and intellectual performance occurring in the early hours of the morning. This happens regardless of any disturbance caused by sleep reduction or deprivation. Task-performance levels can be improved to some extent by practice, by strong motivation and by effort. They can also be affected by personality traits such as introversion and extroversion. It is important to bear in mind that the various systems, once disturbed, recover at different rates, so that while they are still in flux, they are out of step not only with local time but also with each other. Their readjustment and resynchronisation is also dependent on whether the traveller is moving westwards or eastwards. It is well known that recovery from an eastbound flight is more difficult and prolonged than from a westbound one. The time that it takes to recover from jet lag and for the body's rhythms to return to normal also depend to some extent on the individual's adaptability, as well as on his basic health and fitness.

One of the prime factors in the causation of fatigue and tiredness is disturbed sleep, lack of sleep, or inadequate amounts of it. In this situation, an ability to take short naps in which to recover some of that sleep and hence reduce tiredness, is a valuable asset. There are wide differences between different individuals' ability to sleep at times when body and brain chemistry are out of phase with the biological rhythms, but if you can manage to sleep, you can accelerate the return to normal of the disturbed cycles. The use of sleeping tablets, tranquillisers or alcohol to induce sleep in the occasional traveller is of no great moment – all they do, in fact, is prolong the natural process of adaptation. Their use is of great concern, however, when it comes to the air crew, and particularly those in the cockpit.

Bear in mind that **although stimulants such as caffeine in coffee, and amphetamines, help to maintain the performance of even complex tasks during periods of sleep deprivation, they do not remove, but only postpone, the effects of sleep loss. Efficiency is bound to remain reduced, even if you feel as if you are working well.** The sleep that follows the use of such stimulants usually becomes disturbed, and is not as recuperative as it should be.

There is one other kind of stress associated with flying, and that is the stress experienced by those who are frightened of flying, but whose circumstances force them to undergo the ordeal: the businessman who has to travel because of his job, for example, or the person who is pressured into flying to his holiday destination because the rest of the family prefer to go by air.

What can I do to help the situation?

There are certain basic things that you can do in order to reduce the possibility of stress and jet lag, apart from learning specific techniques such as AT in order to deal with specific flight-related anxieties and phobias.

For a start, make sure that you are well organised beforehand, so that you *get plenty of rest or sleep*, and there is no last-minute rush. If you are flying home in a day or two, **do not overexert yourself in unaccustomed physical activity or drink too much alcohol.** Remember that a combination of excessive amounts of alcohol and heat causes marked dehydration – a problem greatly compounded if you have suffered from diarrhoea or vomiting while on holiday. As I said earlier, avoid alcohol during flight, but make sure that you *drink plenty of other fluids*, especially water. And do get as much rest as you can on the plane, particularly if you are on a long flight, no matter how tempting the late-night movie may be!

There are centres that run special relaxation courses for those who are worried about flying, but remember that these are mainly for prophylaxis (prevention), and the techniques must be learned well in advance of your journey. Once a technique such as autogenic training has been learned, it can be used not only to keep down stress and fear levels while you are actually travelling, but also to de-condition you beforehand if you have a severe flying phobia. (See page 135, on *advanced positive affirmations*, and §15.) It is, of course, regular long-distance travellers – and this includes the crew – who can benefit most from AT.

Autogenic training helps to reduce stress at the pre-travel stage, enabling you to cope more efficiently with packing and other preliminaries, for instance, as well as with such problems as delays – for it can be practised anywhere and anytime. It can refresh you before your journey, so that pre-travel tiredness and fatigue become things of the past. Furthermore, it can be practised repeatedly during the flight, helping to alleviate the boredom of the long-haul passenger, as well as enabling both traveller and crew to refresh themselves whenever they want to. Every time the *standard exercises* are practised during the flight they help to bring the body's rhythms and cycles a little nearer to normal, so that the more the exercises are practised the more quickly the body's systems are re-synchronised.

The regular practice of autogenic training after you arrive at your destination not only continues to help restore the body's normal rhythms much more quickly and thereby considerably reduce the effects of jet lag, but also enables you to sleep at will, anywhere and anytime, thus restoring the body's sleep patterns more rapidly and effectively. **In summary, practising AT, before, during and after your journey, is an ideal way of helping the body to function normally when faced with the rigours of long-distance flying.**

§31　Headaches and migraine

Headache is a very common complaint, and migraine is a special version of it. The underlying causes are many, ranging from an infection such as flu or sinusitis to – rarely – a brain tumour, but one of the commonest causes is stress – the so-called tension headache. **If you suffer from chronic or recurrent headaches, or have recently started having migraines, you should always consult your doctor** in order to discover, if possible, the underlying cause. Specific treatments vary, depending on the underlying causes.

What can I do?

Assuming that your headache or migraine has NO UNDERLYING PHYSICAL CAUSE, there is a lot that you can do to reduce both its frequency and its severity.

Diet can be very important. Ensure that you eat well, and have plenty of fresh fruit and vegetables; and take the necessary *supplements* if you suspect that your diet is not adequate. There are a number of foods that can lead to headache, especially migraine, in those who are susceptible. These include citrus fruits (such as oranges), chocolate, over-ripe bananas, cheese, pastry, tomatoes, and fried and fatty foods. Other substances that can have the same effect are coffee and alcohol, especially heavy red wines, port, whisky and brandy, and even beer. So it is very important that you stick to the correct diet, in order to minimise the possible aggravating factors causing your headaches. Also make sure that you take plenty of fluids, especially if the weather is hot or humid.

Other possible contributory factors are *excessive noise, smell, visual strain or glare, or a combination of these.* So try to adjust your environment, where you can, to make life as comfortable as possible for yourself. Make sure that you *get plenty of rest*, as fatigue and tiredness can lead to the onset of headache or migraine. Other significant factors that can contribute to headache are *excitement, anticipation of an important event, change of routine, and overwork;* and, of course, *anxiety, depression, worry and any other kind of stress* that you may be subjected to during your everyday life.

Once the attack has started, you can resort to *standard medications* for relieving the condition, or use *homoeopathic or herbal medicines* such as feverfew. These last can also be used as a preventive measure, to stave off an attack. *Massage* of the head and neck, as well as *osteopathy* and *chiropractic*, can also be of great help, especially if the trigger spot is situated in the neck region.

Autogenic training is particularly important as a preventive measure, because it helps to reduce background stress and thus lessen the possibility of a headache occurring. In addition, the free use of the *offloading exercises* help you to deal with any possible emotional problems. In fact, you can prevent yourself from having headaches or migraine if you practise your AT regularly. The way that you use it in order to control an attack that has just started will vary, depending on the severity as well as on how fast it comes on.

This is what you can do as soon as you feel an attack developing. Sit or lie in a darkened room, and start your *standard exercises*. Repeat 'My neck and shoulders are heavy and warm' or 'My forehead is cool and light (clear)', over and over, until your headache eases or clears up. If your headache starts very quickly, or is particularly severe, then you probably will not at first be able to do the full exercise. In this case, get into an AT position, preferably in a darkened room. Do the scan, and use 'My right (left) arm is heavy' repeatedly. Then, once the headache starts to ease, either go on and do the *full standard AT exercise*, or go straight on to 'My forehead is cool and clear', followed by 'My neck and shoulders are heavy and warm', and repeat them over and over. You will find either that your headache eases immediately, or that you fall asleep and discover that it has gone when you wake up.

If you suffer from severe and prolonged post-migraine lethargy or malaise, you will find that that also will be considerably helped by using AT, especially in the rag-doll or meditative positions.

Remember that, in certain individuals, headache and migraine have a strong connection with repressed and un-resolved emotions, especially anger and sadness. If that is your main poblem, you will find that the *offloading exercises* can be extremely useful, from the point of view of both prevention and recovery once the headache starts. On the other hand, some people actually get a headache *during* an AT exercise. This usually indicates that they are getting in touch with a lot of repressed tensions, feelings and emotions, which will respond well to the offloading exercises, especially the crying and anger ones (lesson 5).

If you find that you cannot prevent or control your headaches or migraine with the standard AT exercises, that also indicates that you have a strong need to offload feelings and emotions – assuming that you have *no underlying serious condition* that could be causing the symptoms. So freely use them (lesson 5), if you are determined both to prevent the pain occurring and to clear it if it does happen again.

Other ways of using AT for the relief of pain are discussed in §42.

§32 Herpes

Herpes infection, of which there are two main types, is caused by a virus. One causes shingles, and the other causes sores around the mouth and in the genital region (and, less commonly, in other parts of the body). Here we are only concerned with the second type of virus. The sores may be single or multiple, and can affect both men and women. The initial infection is often the most serious and painful, and produces the most lesions. Although the virus clears up altogether in some individuals and the infection never recurs, others are subject to recurring attacks which can be very distressing, not only from the point of view of appearance and discomfort but also because of the social implications, especially in the case of genital herpes.

The lesions are often preceded by tingling, burning and pain. These feelings are followed by an inflamed patch which blisters and breaks, and can then get infected by bacteria and form a pussy scab. The lesions are highly infectious, especially in the genital region, and if you are infected you should avoid close personal contact with others, from the time that you feel the lesions starting to about a week after the last has disappeared. If you know you are infected but have no lesions, it is still best to use a condom (sheath) whenever you have intercourse with your partner, in order to prevent the spread of the infection.

There are two very important factors that can precipitate a recurrence: an *inadequate diet*, and *stress* – due either to some other infection or illness, or to social or emotional problems.

What can I do?

The most important thing is, of course, to try to avoid catching the disease. If you do have sex with a casual partner or someone who is infected, **you must use a condom**, even during the remissions, as that does help to some extent. You must also **avoid having sexual or oral contact with the infected person during an attack.**

As already mentioned, *diet* and *nutritional supplements* are very important (see §§5 and 6) There are two important amino acids involved in the herpes infection: lysine, which prevents the virus from growing, and arginine, which enhances the virus's effects and potency. It is therefore advisable to *cut out or minimise your intake of foods containing arginine*, especially if you suffer from recurrent attacks. The most important ones are nuts, seeds and chocolate. But *increase your consumption of foods rich in natural lysine*, which include fresh fish, chicken, milk (cow's and goat's), cheese and mung bean sprouts. Additionally, you can take lysine supplements of up to 1500 mg daily. This amount can be doubled for short periods during an attack.

The sores can be cleaned with any weak antiseptic solution or salt water. Soaking the area in a weak salt solution is not only soothing but can actually help to promote healing. Iodine-based lotions and paints can also be very helpful, both in preventing secondary bacterial infections and in suppressing the herpes virus, as iodine has an anti-viral effect. Don't forget, though, that some people are allergic to iodine. So be careful, and test it first on a small part of the lesion or even on normal skin, before you proceed with painting the whole affected area. Also, there are some very effective *conventional medicines* available, which can reduce not only the duration of an attack but also the recurrence rate. Certain *herbal substances* can be helpful, too. It is best to seek the advice of a qualified herbalist for this.

Since stress has such a detrimental effect on herpes sufferers, *autogenic training* can play a central role in the management of the infection. The *standard exercises* can help in a number of ways. First of all, they not only reduce background stress, but they also enable you to deal positively and effectively with any new stress that may develop. Secondly, they make you aware that there is a great deal that you can do for yourself in order to improve your health and situation; they can reveal to you your own power to manage and heal your condition. The *offloading exercises*, also, can be extremely helpful in dealing with any emotional problems that may be contributing towards the persistence or recurrence of the condition (lesson 5).

Lastly, *positive affirmations* (lessons 9 and 10) can help to alter any negative ideas or attitudes that you may have about yourself, and the use of AT can enhance the healing powers of the mind. Here are some sentences that you can use:

'My —— [affected part] is cool and clear.'
'The lesion does not matter.'
'Herpes infection is immaterial.'
'I am unaffected by the herpes lesions.'
'My lesions heal quickly.'
'My —— is comfortable and healing fast.'
'I know that I can heal my lesions fast.'
'My body has no space for herpes.'

§33 Industry

In today's climate of intense competition, increasing work-loads, high expectations and constant demands for greater productivity all round, people who work in industry, from shop-floor to top management, are subject to enormous amounts of different stresses.

Autogenic training has been used in a variety of industries and in large offices since as long ago as 1943. The main aims in deciding to use the technique have been to increase efficiency, to counterbalance the stresses of long periods of monotonous work, to reduce frustration, aggression and absenteeism, and to enable the individual to deal with the burden of heavy responsibility. Both management and shop-floor workers, in many industries and businesses in England, France and Germany, have benefited. AT has been found to have a great many advantages, in addition to those with which it was originally employed to deal. These advantages – some of them expected and others just unforeseen bonuses – include:

1 The general improvements that are observed in anyone who regularly does AT, such as improved sleeping and ability to relax, plus a reduction in irritability and frustration.
2 Reduction in negative emotional involvement and negative decision-making.
3 Increased ability to cope with long periods of monotonous work more efficiently.
4 Less fatigue and faster recuperation, especially after doing repetitive and boring jobs.
5 Considerable improvement in overall efficiency.
6 Increased ease in learning a new job or function and in assimilating the related knowledge.
7 Increased enjoyment of job and surroundings, often with increased productivity.

8 Increased co-operation between management and workers in trying to improve working conditions, with the aim of reducing to an absolute minimum the stresses associated with the working environment.
9 Increased friendliness and improved communication amongst workers, as well as between workers and management.
10 Less absenteeism.
11 More sustained attention and sharper thinking – during long hours of difficult negotiations, for example.
12 Increased creative initiative.
13 Improvement in both level and duration of concentration.

Apart from the *standard exercises*, which were largely responsible for these beneficial effects, the *offloading exercises* and *positive affirmations* also helped to deal with any underlying emotional problems or frustrations, as well as improving or reinforcing other aspects of the individual's health, wellbeing and efficiency.

This short account demonstrates what an invaluable tool AT can be, in any job or profession, in enabling people to gain the maximum benefits and enjoyment from their work, not only for themselves, but also for those around them.

§34 Infertility

It is a tragedy that at a time when abortions are on the increase, there are couples who are desperate for children but are unable to have any. Infertility can have many causes, attributable to either the man or the woman. It can be as simple as inadequate amounts of sperm in the man, to the obstruction of tubes, or more complicated hormonal problems, in the woman.

It is accepted that **stress and anxiety can be important contributory factors in infertility**. It is well known that many couples manage to conceive soon after they adopt a child or have altogether given up the idea of having children! This probably happens because the anxiety factor is removed from the process of love-making and conception occurs. One factor that helps towards well-being and easier conception is *good nutrition*. Healing can also be very effective.

Autogenic training has been mainly tried with couples who had no underlying physical problems, except that some of the women were shown to have some minor hormonal abnormality known to interfere with fertility. Both partners were taught AT, and it was found that after practising the *standard exercises* a large proportion of the women, even those who had been unable to conceive for as long as ten years, managed to become pregnant. In addition, it was shown that the stress level in both partners was considerably reduced and their relationship improved. The women who conceived found that their pregnancy, delivery and recovery after the birth were greatly helped by AT, as was their bodies' ability to heal – as one would expect from the known facts about AT (§§46 and 48).

It is therefore worthwhile for those couples who are physically normal but unable to conceive, to undertake a course of autogenic training so as to enhance their chances, irrespective of the duration of their unsuccessful attempts.

§35   Irritable bowel syndrome

Unfortunately, this is one of the most common bowel disorders in the West. Although it is of no serious significance in itself, it can make life very uncomfortable and miserable for the sufferer, because of the chronic nature of the symptoms. The commonest is vague abdominal pain, which can affect any part of the abdomen, and the location seems to vary from one time to the next. The pain can be dull and dragging one day, and sharp and colicky the next. The other common symptom is an alteration in the bowel habit, either to constipation or to diarrhoea, and the two can alternate. There is *never* any blood. If you do see blood in your stools, see your doctor immediately, so that he can investigate the cause, as you must in any case for a proper diagnosis.

The real cause of this condition is unknown, but there are a number of contributory factors, which include **insufficient fibre in the diet**, any kind of **bowel infection**, **hormonal disturbances**, **lactose intolerance** (present in milk and dairy products); and, most importantly, **stress**, **anxiety**, **depression** and **personality problems**.

What can I do?

Looking at the possible causes, we can plainly see that there is an enormous amount that you can do to alleviate the problem. First and foremost, your *diet* plays a central role in the management of irritable bowel syndrome. It should be nutritious with plenty of roughage in the way of fruit, vegetables, wholemeal bread, cereals and so on. Avoid alcohol, coffee and strong teas, or reduce them to a minimum, as they seem to aggravate the condition in certain individuals. Preferably, drink herbal teas, especially those that are known to be relaxing, such as camomile, comfrey and fennel. If you have any food allergy or sensitivity, do avoid those foods. Bowel spasms can be alleviated by *proprietary medications*, and by *those prescribed by GPs, homoeopaths and herbalists*.

Autogenic training has a particularly important role to play in the management of this chronic and distressing condition. As in so many other situations, it gives the individual the knowledge and the power to do something positive about it himself. By normalising the functions of the autonomic nervous system (§1) it helps to regulate the bowel again, and thus not only relieves the pain and discomfort but also improves bowel action. The *offloading exercises* (lesson 5) can, of course, be used to deal with any underlying emotional problems that may co-exist. *Positive affirmations* can also help to further alleviate the symptoms. See §24 and §26, for examples of phrases that can be used. And here are some others:

'My bowel functions normally.'
'My bowel is regular and pain-free.'
'My abdomen is warm and comfortable.'

You can make up your own formulae to suit yourself, your problems and your personaltiy, using the guidelines given in lessons 9 and 10.

§36 The menopause

Although about a third of all women, when they reach middle age, have few or no symptoms to do with the cessation of their periods, the other two thirds suffer mild to severe symptoms. Some of these are directly linked with the reduction of female hormones in the body, but others may be related to circumstances, such as a change in the family set-up or other sociologically determined factors. The symptoms can start some time before the periods cease, and can go on for quite a while afterwards. So for those women who have severe symptoms, the period of suffering can be quite considerable.

One of the commonest symptoms is hot flushes, which in a few cases can be associated with sweating. Other symptoms include irritability, moodiness, depression, anxiety, insomnia, weight gain, fluid retention, feeling bloated, aches and pains in muscles or bones, tiredness, loss of concentration, dry vagina, and reduction or total loss of interest in sex. It is advisable to seek the advice of your doctor, particularly if your symptoms are severe, to ensure that there is nothing else, apart from the menopause, that could be contributing to them.

What can I do?

Provided that you are suffering from menopausal symptoms only, it is best to maintain your general fitness by taking plenty of *exercise* and having a *nutritious diet*, with plenty of fresh fruit and vegetables, and *nutritional supplements* including the B group of vitamins – B6 can be particularly important. Minerals that may help are *calcium* and *magnesium*, the former in particular, which can reduce the likelihood of excessive loss of bone (osteoporosis) that can occur at the menopause. Certain *herbal and homœopathic substances* can be beneficial, especially *oil of evening primrose*.

If your symptoms are not helped by any of these, you may require further help from conventional medications, such as *hormone replacement therapy* (HRT). *Psychotherapy* or *counselling* can be helpful if you have personal, family, marital or social problems as well. Therapies such as *reflexology*, *acupuncture* and *massage*, can be of great benefit (see Appendix 1).

The *standard autogenic training exercises* are very helpful in dealing with the kind of stresses that may be present at this time of life, as well as helping you to relax and to cope with any irritability or insomnia. You may find, though, if hot flushes are a problem, that you have to modify the *warmth exercises* by reducing the number of repetitions or by adding 'slightly' to the formula (see lesson 3). You may even have to leave them out altogether, although most women find the warmth exercises quite helpful in the long run. The 'cooling' formulae, particularly 'My forehead is cool and clear', are very helpful during hot flushes. But NEVER use 'cold' or 'very cold', even for short periods, as that can cause unpleasant sensations and side-effects. The *offloading exercises* can be of marked value in dealing with underlying emotional problems (lesson 5), as can the *positive affirmations* for controlling specific symptoms (see lessons 9 and 10).

§37 Menstrual problems

Menstrual problems vary considerably from one woman to the next, and even in the same individual from one time to another, depending on many factors. These can range from age, hormonal problems, infections and inflammations, to stress and emotional troubles, and even shock and change of routine. The commonest symptoms are pain, irregularity and too heavy or too light a bleeding, as well as intermittent bleeding which may be related to having intercourse. Whatever your symptoms, **always seek professional advice**, so that the cause can be ascertained. There are some problems that can only be corrected surgically, but many others can be treated with medication prescribed by a GP, homœopath or herbalist.

What can I do?

Diet and *nutritional supplements* are important, particularly iron replacement if anaemia is present. Once it has been established that there is no serious underlying cause and that the problem is related to stress or emotions, you can do quite a bit to help yourself. The general points to note, and the specific measures to be taken, including the use of *autogenic training*, are basically the same as those described in §§ 5, 6, 36 and 47.

§38   Multiple sclerosis (MS)

The cause of this distressing and often progressive disease
that affects the nervous system is not yet known. The symptoms are extremely varied, depending on which nerve(s) or
part of the nervous system is affected. Two of the commonest
problems, with advanced cases, are tiredness, which may or
may not be related to exertion, and difficulty with walking.

What can I do?

Remember that although there is as yet no treatment that can
cure the disease, stop it in its tracks or slow its progress, there
is usually an immense amount that you can do to improve
your condition, or even reverse it and help yourself return to
almost total normality.

THE RIGHT DIET AND LARGE AMOUNTS OF THE NUTRITIONAL
SUPPLEMENTS THAT ENHANCE THE FUNCTIONING OF BOTH THE
NERVOUS SYSTEM AND THE IMMUNE SYSTEM ARE EXTREMELY
IMPORTANT. The B group of vitamins seem to be particularly
effective (see §§ 5 and 6). It is best to avoid animal fats and
supplement your diet with certain fish and vegetable oils,
especially oil of evening primrose, as they seem to help quite a
number of sufferers. *Massage*, *reflexology*, *osteopathy*,
chiropractic and *spiritual healing* (see Appendix 1), as well as
physiotherapy, *hydrotherapy* and *occupational therapy*, can
all play an important role in improving your condition and
well-being.

It is now generally accepted that the condition of most MS
sufferers is aggravated by stress or by repressed emotions,
either from the past or, more commonly, those deriving from
the problems that the condition imposes on them (and on
their carers, too). *Autogenic training* helps to reduce the
stiffness and spasm of the muscles, particularly those of the
legs, thereby easing mobility. It can also reduce both general

stress and the specific manifestations created by any chronic illness with an uncertain outcome. This uncertainty often causes insecurity, anxiety and frustration; indeed, most individuals with MS have a lot of repressed emotions, resentment and frustration, not least because of the restrictions that the disease imposes on their lives. The *offloading exercises* can be of immense value, as these troublesome emotions often seem to be locked up in the limb muscles. A number of MS sufferers that I have known have found that the combination of the *standard exercises* and the offloading exercises has improved their walking significantly – even dramatically, in a few cases. *Positive affirmations* can be very helpful in enabling the sufferer to cope effectively with more specific symptoms (see lessons 9 and 10).

There seem to be quite a number of people, especially women, who develop MS phobia, and as a consequence experience symptoms of aching, pins and needles and even weakness in their arms and legs. The condition of these individuals does not seem to be helped by negative investigation results and repeated reassurances. However, they often seem to respond dramatically, with the complete disappearance of their symptoms, once they use AT in all its aspects, particularly the *offloading exercises* (lesson 5). In my experience, almost all of these people appear to have repressed some powerful emotion or memory into their limbs. When they become aware of this and deal with it as described elsewhere in this book (lesson 5), their symptoms often seem to melt away.

§39 Muscle disorders

Stiffness, aching, pain and soreness can appear in any muscular or bony part of the body. Although the symptoms may occur for no apparent reason, there can be many and varied underlying causes, including local disease or a reaction to a general or widespread disease which needs to be investigated. One contributory factor which must always be borne in mind is **stress**, and **strong emotions** which may have been repressed into that particular area or group of muscles. Repression of anger, sadness and so on into muscles and joints is very common (see §§16 and 18). The resulting pain or stiffness can be quite disabling, though there may not be any underlying physical condition. The repression need not be of emotional origin. It could have associations with a past injury, trauma or operation, the psychological pain or other aspects of which were not worked through at the time. This kind of problem may become particularly noticeable during the AT exercises, as what we call *discharges* (§2).

So-called 'rheumatic pains' for which no physical cause can be found – whether or not they are related to changes in the weather – seem to settle spontaneously with the regular practice of the *standard AT exercises*. Once the trainee has realised that the pains are related to a past trauma, if that is indeed the case, the 'rheumatism' seems to disappear, as do the pain, soreness and stiffness. Other conditions that seem to be particularly amenable to treatment by AT are fibrositis, lumbago and torticollis – a condition in which the muscles of the neck go into spontaneous spasm, usually quite painful (§59).

Diet and *nutritional supplements* are also quite important (see §§ 5 and 6). *Massage*, with or without oils (*aromatherapy*), *osteopathy* and *chiropractic* (see Appendix 1), as well as *physiotherapy, hydrotherapy, conventional, homoeopathic and herbal medicines*, can all play an important part.

Apart from the *standard exercises*, the frequent use of the *offloading exercises* (lesson 5), especially the anger and crying ones, can be invaluable in the relief of these conditions. *Positive affirmations* can also be used in order to enhance the healing effects of AT. This can include applying warmth or heaviness formulae to the affected part. Try:

'My —— [affected part] is warm (and/or heavy).'

You can, of course, make up your own phrases to suit your own symptoms. You can also consult other sections, such as the one on arthritis (§16) and the one on backache (§18), for other affirmations.

§40 Myalgic encephalomyelitis (ME or post-viral syndrome)

This chronic and distressing condition, although first mentioned as long ago as the 1950s, has only relatively recently been recognised as a serious clinical syndrome. Although the symptoms often appear after an influenza-like infection, in some people myalgic encephalomyelitis seems to start for no apparent reason, except that usually it seems to be related to periods of stress or emotional disturbance.

The symptoms vary in intensity, depending on the severity of the condition and on which body systems are primarily affected. The commonest and longest-lasting seem to be lack of concentration, excessive sleepiness, weakness and pain in the muscles, and extreme tiredness and lethargy. Of these, the last three are usually the most prominent and distressing. The illness usually follows a chronic course, lasting from a few months to a few years, and although there is no known conventional medical treatment for it at present, there is an enormous amount that you can do to help yourself, not only to shorten its duration but also to overcome it altogether.

What can I do?

First of all, *complete rest* is essential during the acute phase. You must also have plenty of rest during the recovery period, and not let yourself get over-tired. Once the acute phase is over and you start feeling better, as with all chronic debilitating conditions that affect the immune system (see §§ 13, 21 and 48) you must *build up your general fitness* through graduated amounts of exercise. Keep within your capabilities, and don't over-exert yourself. *Diet* and *nutritional supplements* are extremely important (§§ 5 and 6), as are certain *herbs* and homoeopathic remedies that build up the body and the immune system. It is best to consult a qualified herbalist or homœopath to get further information on these.

Massage has health-enhancing properties, as apart from anything else it makes you feel good and relaxed. *Reflexology* and *acupuncture* (see Appendix 1) may also have a place in some people's treatment. **Stress**, **anxiety** and **depression** have been shown to be implicated both in the inception of the condition and in its perpetuation. Furthermore, the various manifestations of myalgic encephalomyelitis can in themselves be very stressful and cause emotional problems for both sufferer and carers – not least the stress associated with a chronic condition of uncertain cause and progress. Many sufferers were thought to be malingerers before the condition was properly recognised, and the carers have to cope not only with all this uncertainty in someone they love, but also with the physical act of looking after an individual who may be disabled in both physical and emotional terms, sometimes severely.

Autogenic training can be extremely beneficial here, as not only does it help to reduce background stress but it also helps you to become much more positive in your outlook and to become aware that there is a lot that you can do for yourself to improve the situation. This knowledge, and the fact that you will be able to empower yourself to fight the disease, is a crucial factor in speeding up the recovery process.

The *offloading exercises* (lesson 5) can be of immense value in enabling you to deal not only with the deep repressed emotions that may have helped to trigger the illness, but also with all the emotions and frustrations that are stirred up when it starts. When you use these exercises, though, be gentle with yourself. Do them within your own physical capabilities and modify them to suit your needs. Please do make sure, though, that you do them, as they can considerably speed up your recovery.

Other symptoms can be further alleviated by the use of *positive affirmations* (fully covered in lessons 9 and 10 and in §§ 21, 25, 38 and 48). Try these phrases, too:

'I am full of energy and vitality.'
'I am healing myself.'
'I am strong, healthy and full of energy.'
'My concentration is as sharp as ever.'

'My concentration is normal.'
'I concentrate as well as ever.'

Again, I give just a few examples. You can make up your own phrases, or use any of those given elsewhere in the book, that seem to suit your specific needs.

§41 Obesity

Obesity can be defined as an increase of more than 10 per cent over the normal expected weight, taking into account height, age and build. Although the commonest cause is eating in excess of the body's requirements, there are some specific medical conditions that can also lead to obesity. It is therefore advisable to make sure that there is no such underlying medical condition, especially if obesity has developed suddenly and recently.

What can I do?

The central factor in losing weight is MOTIVATION! *Diet*, of course, is of paramount importance, and the number of calories taken in must depend on the amount of energy that needs to be put out; a heavy manual worker, for instance, requires a lot more calories than an office worker. Restriction of fluids is important, as body fat tends to act rather like a sponge and absorb fluid, causing a feeling of bloatedness as well as increasing weight. When calculating your total calorie intake, *do include alcohol*, if you drink it. Some people insist on taking appetite-suppressant drugs in order to help them lose weight. This is a very dangerous thing to do, as most of these drugs either have unpleasant side-effects or are addictive, or both. Some herbal and vegetable remedies can be quite helpful, especially in producing bulk, thus filling up the stomach and depressing the desire to eat. It is best to consult a qualified herbalist or dietician for these.

PLEASE DO NOT attend slimming clinics that mainly use appetite-suppressants and/or diuretics (fluid-reducing drugs in the form of tablets or injections). In combination they can be very dangerous to your long-term health, especially if there is no proper supervision by a qualified medical practitioner.

Exercise is very important, not only for maintaining general well-being but also to increase energy output and to burn off extra calories and fat.

Autogenic training can be helpful in a number of ways. First, some people eat excessively when they are under stress. By reducing the general stress level, AT controls that aspect of over-eating. Then, it has been shown that some people start to over-eat or indulge in sweet or fattening foods when they get anxious or depressed. Here the *offloading exercises* (lesson 5), which permit the individual to cope with his or her unresolved emotions, can be of tremendous value. Finally, one of the most helpful AT tools in the management of obesity is the *positive affirmations* (lessons 9 and 10). But they can be quite difficult to use in this context. What is needed is a careful appraisal of the situation; you must work out *why* you are overweight. Phrases such as 'I'll lose weight' are totally inadequate. Instead, ask yourself whether, for instance, you are eating too much at each meal. Are you eating too many meals? Are you eating in between meals? Or do you eat too many chocolates? Once you have worked out what your problem is, then you can make up a formula to suit your needs – which, incidentally, can vary from time to time, and so you may have to change your phrases accordingly.

I had one man in one of my groups whose obesity was largely caused by an addiction to chocolates. Every time he went past a chocolate shop he had to go in and buy pounds of them. He even had to resort to planning his routes so as to avoid passing any chocolate shops! But using the affirmation, 'I am indifferent to chocolates', he managed to break his addiction so thoroughly that he could even resist an opened box of chocolates placed beside him.

One problem that you must be aware of when using AT affirmations for losing weight is that, quite unlike other affirmations, weight-losing sentences can lose their effect very quickly and may have to be changed every week or so, in order to remain maximally effective. Here are a few examples. Don't forget that you can make up your own to suit your needs and personality (see also §§27 and 28).

'I know I can stick to my diet.'
'I'll eat less at each meal.'

'I'll refrain from eating between meals.'
'My diet is fun and enjoyable.'
'It is easy to follow my diet.'
'Others may over-eat, but I won't.'
'Small meals are adequate for me.'
'Small meals are filling and satisfying.'
'I won't eat between meals.'

§42 Pain and itching

Itching is a sensation that is caused by the irritation of specific nerve endings in the skin, which may result from both external and internal irritants. The nervous pathway that carries this sensation to the brain is very close to that which carries the pain sensation, and this is probably why a severe itching sensation can sometimes seem painful at the same time.

Pain is one of the commonest and most distressing symptoms. It is interesting that the pain threshold varies dramatically from one individual to the next, and even occasionally in the same individual from one time to the next, depending on a number of factors. So the perception of pain is very subjective; what may be agonising to one person may be but a slight annoyance to another. The most important factors towards exacerbation of pain can be fear, anxiety, depression, anger and uncertainty about the possible cause.

Pain is not only physical. It can also be psychological, emotional or even spiritual. THIS DOES NOT MEAN THAT THE SUFFERER IS IMAGINING IT. Far from it – the pain is real enough. What it does mean, though, is that its origin goes back to some past unresolved or repressed emotion or memory. Repressed into the unconscious, the emotion later comes out in a modified physical form such as a painful back or arthritis.

I personally suffered a great deal of this kind of pain for some years, before I became aware of the nature of it and dealt with it through AT. I was diagnosed as having some form of 'arthritis' which affected most of my joints, but particularly my neck and back, as a result of which I had to resort to wearing a neck collar and a spinal corset, as well as having to take anti-inflammatory drugs and pain-killers. These drugs produced a severe inflammation of the stomach, so I was then given others to heal that. I was a walking psychosomatic disaster, unable to come off any of the drugs.

However, within a few months of doing AT regularly, practising the offloading exercises freely and having analytical therapy, my symptoms settled down, and not only was I able to discard the collar and the corset but I was also able gradually to come off all the medications. I have never felt as fit as I do now. I take only an occasional pain-killer, and if I feel any of the old pains starting up again I know that all I have to do is concentrate more on my standard AT exercises IN CONJUNCTION WITH THE OFFLOADING EXERCISES, and the symptoms disappear pretty quickly. This is, of course, a personal experience, and it may not be exactly the same for you.

Pain is your body's way of telling you that something is not quite right. So listen to it, and find out what the cause of your problem may be. Then you can try to do something about it. If the underlying cause can be removed, you will get rid of that particular pain. So consult your GP for assessment and diagnosis. However, if the cause of your pain cannot be immediately removed, then you may have to resort to *conventional, or herbal or homœopathic, remedies*. Techniques that may work for specific conditions include *reflexology, osteopathy, chiropractic, physiotherapy, hydrotherapy, massage, touch therapy* and *spiritual healing*. (See Appendix 1.) If your pain does not respond to any of these, including AT, you can be referred by your doctor to a pain clinic which specialises in intractable pains.

Autogenic training has a very important role to play in the context of pain. For a start, by helping to reduce or even abolish background stress, it reduces muscle spasm and tension, which can be quite a significant source of pain. In addition to the *standard exercises*, the *offloading exercises* can be very helpful, if the pain is aggravated by emotional factors. The way that AT works in trying to deal with pain and itching is quite different from most other techniques, insofar as you do not confront the pain or itching, as this can in itself exacerbate it by adding another layer of stress to an already stressful situation. In other words, rather than aggravating the problem by actively concentrating on it, adopt a *passive attitude*. By doing this you will cut down the number of pain-producing stimuli, whether internal or external, reaching the brain, and thereby reduce your perception of pain. AT thus helps to dissolve, or considerably reduce, the psychological manifestations of pain, irrespective of whether there are any underlying physical causes.

Depending on the severity of the pain, autogenic training can be used in a number of different ways. If you are in a great deal of pain, you may find it impossible to do the full standard exercises immediately. So try the *short exercise* (lesson 1) repeatedly. You will find either that this permits you to dissociate yourself from the pain sufficiently, or that the pain diminishes enough for you to be able to go on and do the *full AT exercises*. Sometimes you may find that just doing the short exercise or 'My neck and shoulders are heavy' (lesson 2) will be sufficient to free you from the pain, so that you can then continue with your daily routine. The short exercise can also be a valuable tool in dealing with difficult and potentially painful situations, such as having dental treatment or other surgery without a general anaesthetic. It helps to get you fully relaxed, and in so doing reduces the pain and enables you to cope with the situation much more effectively.

I know many people who were petrified of going to the dentist before undertaking their AT training, but who afterwards not only found it easy to go, but were even able to have their treatment without a local anaesthetic! I certainly DO NOT recommend this to the novice, as you must be very experienced in getting into very deep AT states to be able to do it. It is interesting, though, that the effect is totally different from that experienced during hypnosis, in which you are usually unaware of the pain. In AT, you are aware of the pain and discomfort but you totally dissociate from it, and so it does not seem to affect you.

Once you are able to get into deep states of AT, YOU WILL FIND THAT YOU ARE ABLE TO DISSOCIATE FULLY from uncomfortable, itchy or painful areas of your body, at least for the duration of the AT state. And often you will be able to overcome the pain or itching, or at least a substantial part of it, by regular practice. This is one reason why AT is so useful for those suffering from serious diseases such as cancer or AIDS, as they can dissociate from their distress at least while they are in their AT state; and once they come out of it, they can cope with their problems much more adequately.

As I have pointed out before in this book, it is well known that stress and repressed or unresolved emotions or memories can not only cause pain but also exacerbate and perpetuate it. So if there *are* any such feelings or memories that may be contributing towards your symptoms, the *offloading exercises* (lesson 5) can be of immense help. It is well worth trying any and all of them at different times, as you may often be totally unaware of what the underlying feeling, emotion or memory actually is. In certain painful conditions such as migraine the emotions may be easier to decipher, since they are often associated with repressed anger. The offloading exercises that seem to be particularly effective in the relief of pain are the *humming and moaning exercises* (pages 91 and 97).

Positive affirmations (lessons 9 and 10) can also help to deal with pain. It is important to bear in mind, though, that for this purpose we do not usually concentrate on the painful area during our AT exercises. We tend to use the words 'warmth', 'heaviness' or 'cooling' as usual, but we use 'it' – as in 'It feels comfortable' – instead of specifying the affected part. For the use of specific positive affirmations, see, for instance, §§ 16, 18, 24, 31, 35, 39, 49 and 59. Here are a few other examples:

'Pain is immaterial. I feel comfortable.'
'It feels pain-free (itch-free) and comfortable.'
'I am strong, healthy and pain-free (itch-free).'
'I am healing myself.'
'I free myself of any pain (itch) or distress.'
'I am unaffected by pain (itching).'
'My body and mind relieve me of pain (itching).'
'I allow my being to free itself of pain (itching) and distress.'
'I permit myself to work through the pain (itching).'
'As I relax, the pain (itching) floats out of my body.'
'I have no need for pain (itch).'

For these three affirmations, actually take your mind to the painful or itchy area (see lesson 10):

'My —— [affected part] is cool (warm, heavy) [depending on what feels right].'
'My —— [affected part] is cool.' (This one is especially for itching.)
'My —— [affected part] is pain-free (itch-free).'

§43 Palpitations

What are palpitations? People who suffer from them have different conceptions of what the term means. The commonest meaning is a rapid, but regular, heart rate, either constant or intermittent. Others say that they have palpitations only if their heartbeat is forceful and they can hear it; it is not necessarily fast. Yet others complain of palpitations only when their heartbeat is irregular. This may mean an occasional dropped beat, or it may be totally irregular.

Although most of these kinds of palpitation can be caused by a sympathetic overreaction to anxiety, emotions and other stresses, there are many other possible causes as well, so if you think that you are suffering from palpitations, before you put it down to anxiety or stress **get yourself fully checked over by your doctor**.

What can I do?

There are many things that you can do in order to reduce the likelihood of this uncomfortable symptom occurring. For a start, *avoid coffee, strong tea and any other caffeine-containing drink*, as caffeine can both cause and perpetuate palpitations, as can *alcohol* and *tobacco*. So try to avoid these as well. Some herbal teas can be very relaxing, such as camomile, comfrey and fennel, as well as herbal remedies (see a qualified herbalist). *Conventional drug therapy* can also play quite an important role, especially when there is an underlying physical or medical condition.

Once again, *autogenic training* is very useful in reducing background stress and in cutting down the production of stress-related hormones, and this in turn helps to reduce both the rate and the force of the heartbeats. However, occasionally the use of the phrase 'My heartbeat is calm and regular' (lesson 4) can actually exacerbate the situation, particularly if there is a lot of anxiety stored at the heart level. In this situation it is best either to avoid the phrase or to introduce it gradually and gently. And certainly, if your palpitations are of the kind characterised by an irregular heartbeat, do avoid the phrase altogether. The *offloading exercises* are, of course, extremely important, particularly those associated with the release of anxiety and anger, as we carry an enormous amount of repressed emotion at the heartbeat level. Please **do not experiment with phrases to do with the heart and circulation**. But you can use *positive affirmations* such as:

'My heartbeat is calm and comfortable.'
'My heartbeat is slow and regular.'

§44 Parkinson's disease

This is an insidious and chronic disease, which usually starts late in life because of a disturbance of certain chemicals in the brain. It can, though, start suddenly as the result of an accident involving the brain or as a side-effect of certain drugs. The main symptoms are usually spasm and stiffness of the muscles, with a 'pill-rolling' tremor of the hands. Emotional problems such as depression can also occur.

What can I do?

Although there is no cure, there is a lot that the sufferer and his family and friends can do in order to improve both his health and the outlook as far as the progression of the condition is concerned.

First, make sure that you follow the general health guidelines as regards your *diet, nutritional supplements* and *exercise* (§§ 5 and 6). *Healing, massage, reflexology, physiotherapy, osteopathy* and *chiropractic* can all help to alleviate muscle stiffness and prevent the stiffness of the joints that may follow. *Spiritual healing* can be of tremendous help to some individuals. There are now *conventional medicines* that can help to reduce both the stiffness and the tremor, although unfortunately some of them produce quite marked side-effects in some people.

Although, as far as we know, *autogenic training* cannot restore the balance of chemicals in the brain, it can help enormously in a number of ways. Apart from reducing background stress and anxiety, which can aggravate the condition, AT can help via the use of the *standard exercises*, especially the *warmth exercise* for the limbs, to alleviate considerably the stiffness of the muscles. It can also help to improve concentration and to prevent the progression of the disease. It has been found that a number of patients, by practising AT, have been able to substantially reduce their intake of medications, thereby reducing the side-effects that they had previously suffered. A few actually managed to come off the drugs altogether.

The *offloading exercises* (lesson 5) can help you to deal with the emotional problems that may be associated with the condition, and the *positive affirmations* can enable you to control specific symptoms (lessons 9 and 10). See also §§16, 18, 25, 27 and 39.

§45   Phantom limb syndrome

This refers to the pain that occurs at the site of a non-existent limb which has been traumatically lost through accident or surgery. It can also occur as spasms in the paralysed limbs of paraplegics who have no other sensations in their legs. How and why this sort of pain occurs is not very clear, especially since it does not seem to be helped by any particular treatment. As the pain can be very severe, chronic and intractable, it can be extremely distressing and depressing to the sufferer. I believe that many pains are repressed into tissues, organs, and so on, as a result of trauma – irrespective of the cause. Much of the problem with this condition may have to do with the sufferer not having resolved the emotional pain that resulted from the accident or surgery at the time; and this is what he or she is experiencing at a conscious level in the paralysed or non-existent limb(s). It may partly explain why the condition is so resistant to standard methods of pain control, including nerve blocks.

Autogenic training is very helpful in reducing the sufferer's general stress level as well as that specifically to do with his or her condition. And as the body relaxes, the attacks of spastic pain seem to lessen considerably, and even sometimes disappear. I have found that the symptoms can be greatly alleviated by the *offloading exercises* in association with the *standard AT exercises. Positive affirmations* can also be helpful (lessons 9 and 10). Try:

'The pain does not matter.'
'My leg (arm) stump is pain-free.'

Others can be used to suit your general situation and the location of the pain, especially those mentioned in §42 on pain relief.

If when practising autogenic training you find that the symptoms in the affected limb get worse, it may be worth excluding that part of the body from the standard exercises at first. You can then gradually incorporate it again as the symptoms ease.

§46 Pregnancy, labour and delivery

Pregnancy should be a happy state. Unfortunately, and for a variety of reasons, it is not always the case. This may have to do with the emotional, psychological or social problems of the mother, or with the physical symptoms that the pregnancy may produce, which are often related to the increased levels of hormones in the body during this natural physiological state. Complaints of pregnancy include nausea, vomiting, constipation, insomnia, shortness of breath, irritability, tension and anxiety, indigestion and physical discomfort, especially during the later stages.

What can I do?

First, ensure that you are as fit as possible, by taking *regular exercise* and following a *good, nutritious diet*, with plenty of fresh fruit and vegetables. Your requirement of *nutritional supplements*, particularly *iron and folic acid*, increases considerably at this time, since the baby too requires these essential constituents for its growth and development. Avoid smoking at all costs. *Massage*, *reflexology* and *hydrotherapy* (exercise in water) can all be useful in reducing muscle tension and thus promoting a feeling of well-being in the mother. The old adage that happy babies are born to happy mothers seems to run true.

Autogenic training brings benefits in all three of the main stages: in the antenatal period, during delivery, and in the postnatal period.

THE ANTENATAL STAGE

It is important that you start to use AT as soon as possible in pregnancy. It has been found that the *standard exercises* help to reduce or even abolish many of the minor symptoms listed above. Also, by reducing tension and stress, as well as blood pressure and heart rate, AT helps to prevent the onset of toxaemia of pregnancy, one of the most serious complications for both mother and baby. One of the main aims of antenatal care is to prevent toxaemia developing.

IT IS IMPORTANT TO MODIFY, OR EVEN OMIT, SOME OF THE STANDARD FORMULAE, ESPECIALLY THOSE DEALING WITH WARMTH IN THE LIMBS AND THE SOLAR PLEXUS, IF YOU FIND THAT YOU ARE GETTING PALPITATIONS OR BECOMING TOO WARM DURING THE EXERCISES. This is quite common and nothing to worry about, since both circulation and heartbeat are increased in pregnancy anyway, to allow for the development of the baby. Any further increase in circulation brought on by the warmth exercises can be uncomfortable, so if this does happen either reduce the number of repetitions or add the word 'slightly' to 'warm' – or even, as I have said, leave out any troublesome exercises altogether (lessons 4 and 7). Don't worry, if you have to do this, that your AT will be ineffective. You will still be able to get the full benefits as long as you use the other phrases regularly and frequently.

Also, the *offlanding exercises* can as usual be of immense value in dealing with any underlying emotional problems that may be present (such as unwanted pregnancy, mental disharmony and so on) and the readjustments that need to be addressed.

THE DELIVERY STAGE

The *full standard exercises* can be practised regularly and frequently during labour, especially the first stage. They will help you to relax, and in so doing allow the body to co-ordinate the various physiological activities involved, so that the whole procedure of delivery and birth can proceed much more effectively, irrespective of the type of delivery that you decide on. AT will help you to refresh yourself whenever you need to, so that fatigue and exhaustion are kept at bay. It will also help to keep blood pressure, heart rate and respiration in check, and by reducing stress, tension and muscle spasm will minimise any pain. At the same time, by regulating and co-ordinating the movements of the uterus AT will increase the effectiveness of the contractions, thereby probably shortening labour – provided, of course, that there are no physical obstructions to the outlet of the pelvis. These beneficial effects also help the baby to fare better, making it less likely to suffer foetal distress during its passage through the birth canal.

It is assumed here that the antenatal care and delivery have been properly supervised by a doctor or qualified midwife, so that there are no physical problems that could interfere with the proper functioning of the womb and the birth canal. AT should only be used to assist and ease the normal healthy processes.

If you do your exercises in such a way that the phrase 'It breathes me' coincides with the height of the contraction, all well and good. But if, like most trainees, you find that quite difficult to do, you may find the frequent use of the *short exercise* or 'My neck and shoulders are heavy' during the contractions very helpful. If you do this, though, it is important to do the *full standard exercises* as well as the *neck and shoulders exercises* in between contractions, in order to refresh yourself and prevent the onset of fatigue and exhaustion.

It has been found that a great many women notice a considerable reduction in pain and duration of the second stage of delivery using the above method. A few have even said that, using their AT regularly and frequently, they experienced no pain during this stage.

THE POSTNATAL STAGE

It is well known, and often mentioned in this book, that AT helps to speed up markedly the healing processes of the body (§48). Consequently, its regular practice after delivery is extremely effective in promoting recovery from the traumas, physical, emotional and psychological, that may have been inflicted on the mother. AT helps to boost the production of milk and to reduce the likelihood of postnatal emotional disturbances, including depression – often referred to as 'baby blues'. The *offloading exercises* can be immensely valuable should this happen. Another bonus of using AT is that insomnia is less likely to be a problem. The mother usually finds that she is able to go straight back to sleep again after getting up to attend to the baby, as well as being able to refresh herself during the day by doing regular exercises and using the *neck and shoulders exercises*. And the *positive affirmations* can be of great benefit if some specific problem such as retention of placenta and urine or post-operative pain develops (see §§ 62, 48, 42). All in all, AT is an immensely effective tool in improving and normalising all aspects of pregnancy and delivery.

§47 Pre-menstrual syndrome (PMS)

Pre-menstrual syndrome (or tension) is an unpleasant, recurring condition that affects up to 50 per cent of women,
especially between the ages of thirty and forty. The symptoms
vary considerably from person to person, but they usually
include fluid retention, breast discomfort or even swelling,
anxiety, depression and other symptoms of either over- or
underactivity of the autonomic nervous system. (§1). The
severity of the symptoms also varies considerably, and in
extreme cases the psychological manifestations can lead to
antisocial, or even criminal, behaviour. Even in women with
only moderate symptoms, the worry and fear of their getting
worse can make their lives a misery.

What can I do?

Make sure that you have *plenty of exercise*, as well as a
nutritious diet, with plenty of fresh fruit and vegetables.
Nutritional supplements (§§ 5 and 6), especially vitamin B6,
magnesium and oil of evening primrose, can be of
tremendous benefit. As some symptoms are due to fluid
retention, it may be advisable to *restrict your fluid intake* to a
maximum of two pints a day during the period that you
normally suffer from PMS. As fat absorbs and retains large
amounts of fluid, it may be a good idea to lose weight if you
are overweight. Using *conventional, herbal or homœopathic
medications* in order to get rid of excessive fluids can also be
helpful.

   A great many PMS symptoms are due to an imbalance of
hormones and of the autonomic nervous system; *autogenic
training* can be quite effective in helping to correct these
imbalances, thereby alleviating the condition. Practising the
standard exercises will lead to self-regulating and healing, and
any minor hormonal problems will tend to normalise. The
symptoms of sympathetic overactivity, such as palpitations,

tremor, anxiety, irritability and insomnia, are also likely to be relieved. Stress often exacerbates the symptoms, and you can control that, and thus alleviate the symptoms, with the standard exercises. Don't forget the *offloading exercises* (lesson 5), which can be so helpful in dealing with repressed or unworked-through emotions, feelings or memories. You can also use *positive affirmations* to control specific symptoms if you have not obtained adequate relief from any of the above (lessons 9 and 10, and see also §§ 36 and 37).

§48 Recovery after illness, surgery and accident

Illness in general, and surgery and accident in particular, are traumatic and stressful, causing a lot of anxiety and fear as well as pain. All this may reduce or interfere with the healing powers of the body. *Autogenic training*, which can be beneficial both before and after surgery as well as after illness or accident, is purpose-made for this situation.

It is important to realise, though, that in order for the body to heal quickly and effectively it must be in a healthy state, and so you must keep yourself generally fit by doing *regular exercise* and eating *nutritious food*, as well as taking any *supplements* that may be necessary for your own particular needs. The intake of vitamin C should be considerably increased in order to speed up the healing of wounds (§6). From the preventive point of view, doing your AT regularly will help you to avoid falling sick too readily. If you do become ill, you can use all aspects of your AT to speed up your recovery (for which you should consult the sections on specific conditions). Preoperatively, AT helps you to relax and to deal with the anxiety, fear or other emotional problems that may precede any kind of surgery, no matter how minor. You are then able to face the surgery in a much better frame of mind, which in turn will permit you to recover more quickly and thoroughly.

The *standard AT exercises* have been shown to improve the whole process of healing and normalising within the body after surgery. This applies even if your immune system is deficient. AT has also been shown to reduce muscle tension and pain at or around the operation site. You can further supplement the healing powers of AT by using the *offloading exercises*. Do make sure, though, to adjust them according to your physical disability (lesson 5). *Positive affirmations* (lessons 9 and 10) are also helpful here.

There are many recorded cases that demonstrate AT's

beneficial effects on people's healing powers. Here is what happened to one of my own trainees.

This sixty-two-year-old woman had been practising AT for about six months when she developed an acute inflammation of the bowel (diverticulitis), which led to its perforation. The perforation was demonstrated by X-rays. As normally happens in these cases, she was rested, as was her bowel by drip-feeding her. When she was X-rayed again after forty-eight hours no sign of a perforation was found, and as she felt well she was discharged. Within a week of having been admitted to hospital she felt well enough to start playing tennis again! During the whole of her stay in hospital she had done her AT regularly, and further enhanced its effects by using positive healing affirmations.

This episode demonstrates the close harmony that can be achieved between traditional treatment and AT in order to speed up the healing and recovery processes. However, it is *extremely important* to bear in mind what has already been emphasised several times in this book – **that AT should be used only in conjunction with other techniques, including surgery, which may be an essential or even life-saving part of treatment.**

§49 Sciatica

At its worst, this is one of the most painful conditions from which anyone can suffer. It usually affects one leg, and is caused by the irritation or inflammation of the sciatic nerve, which extends from the lower back to the foot. Consequently, depending on the severity of the condition, the pain can extend from the lower back as far as the foot. There are many possible causes, and it is always advisable to see your GP if it does not improve quickly, to find out what is causing it. Some treatments are specific to certain causes; **bear in mind that treating the condition in the wrong way can be extremely hazardous**.

What can I do?

Once you know the cause of your sciatica, and provided that there is NO SERIOUS UNDERLYING PHYSICAL CAUSE, there is quite a lot that you can do in order to relieve your symptoms and improve your general condition. In the acute phase, when the symptoms can be very severe and disabling, you may find *rest* and *pain-killers* very helpful. *Massage* with or without oils and creams, as well as *heat* in the form of hot water bottles, hot baths or an infra-red lamp, are also beneficial. In less severe or more chronic cases (provided that there are NO PHYSICAL ABNORMALITIES), *physiotherapy, cranial osteopathy, osteopathy, chiropractic* and *hypnotherapy* can considerably shorten the period of disability and suffering.

Autogenic training can play a very valuable part in the more chronic cases, probably because the symptoms are often partly due to repressed tension in the muscles of the back and legs. The *standard exercises* can be used to reduce this kind of background stress. However, you will at first have to modify the rag-doll (or simple sitting) position (page 48) if you find it impossible to get into that position, especially if you have undergone surgery, for instance. You will find, though, that with practice and as time goes by and the tension level in your back muscles drops, you will be able to use this position and will even find it quite soothing and helpful. A great many of my trainees have been able to discard the spinal corset, which they sometimes have to wear if the condition is very severe, after using AT for a few months. Since people who suffer from sciatica often seem to have repressed enormous amounts of emotion, especially sadness and anger, into the affected areas, the *offloading exercises* can be particularly effective. *Positive affirmations* (lessons 9 and 10) can also be very helpful. (See also §§16, 18, 39 and 42.)

§50 Sexual problems

Sexual problems (dysfunctions) in both men and women can have a great many underlying physical as well as psychological causes, which must be investigated. Male symptoms include hasty emission, premature ejaculation, functional disturbance such as loss of erection prior to penetration, and inability to ejaculate during coitus. Common symptoms in women are vaginal spasm, painful intercourse and frigidity. Provided that there is no physical cause and that the symptoms are mainly related to anxiety and other psychological or emotional problems, a *combination of sex education, counselling and therapy* (if needed), *and autogenic training* has been found to be helpful in relieving and overcoming these problems.

What can I do?

As far as AT is concerned, you may use just the *standard exercises* to help relieve background stress and anxiety. But you may find that the *positive affirmations* (lessons 9 and 10) can enhance the normalising effects of AT and thereby reduce the symptoms. Here are a few examples:

'My erection is strong and maintained.'
'I know that I'll hold my erection on penetration.'
'My orgasm is slow and delayed.'
'My ejaculation is delayed.'
'I don't ejaculate spontaneously.'
'I enjoy being inside my partner.'
'My erection will hold while I enter my partner.'
'I enjoy sex.'
'Sex is pleasurable and satisfying.'
'I know that I can satisfy my partner.'
'I am gentle and loving with my partner.'
'I know that I can delay my orgasm.'

'I enjoy making love, and being made love to.'
'I am turned on by my partner.'
'I enjoy making love to my partner.'
'His/her touch and foreplay turns me on.'
'I feel sexy towards my partner.'
'I can hold back my orgasm.'
'My orgasm is delayed.'
'I know that I enjoy having sex.'
'My vagina is free and painless.'
'My vulva/vagina is warm (heavy, cool).'
'I want him inside me.'
'I relax and enjoy penetration.'
'I enjoy being penetrated.'

§51 Skin ailments

Eczema, psoriasis and urticaria are three of the commonest as well as most distressing skin disorders, and affect a very large proportion of the population. Apart from the fact that they are unsightly and cause social rejection and stress, especially in children, they are also often irritating and distressing, and keep the sufferers awake at night. The causes of these conditions are unknown, but allergies, sensitivities, stress and emotional problems play a very important part in both their inception and their persistence and exacerbation.

What can I do?

Diet can be very important, especially if an element of allergy or sensitivity is involved. You must eat good, nutritious food, with, as always, plenty of fresh fruit and vegetables. And be sure to avoid the things that you may be allergic to, if you know what they are. It may be necessary to consult an allergist or nutritionist to determine what substances, either locally or generally, are contributing towards the symptoms. Once that has been established, it may then be possible to desensitise you against those substances (allergens) that are causing the allergy.

Supplements such as zinc and selenium, which improve general health and immunity, can be quite important, as can oil of evening primrose, especially if you suffer from eczema. If you think that you may be allergic to soap or detergents, DO AVOID THEM. The so-called biological washing powders which contain enzymes are notorious for causing all forms of skin rashes. Some people are even allergic to the soda that is commonly present even in non-biological detergents. You must avoid this as well if you suffer from any skin rashes. Locally applied *ointments* and *creams*, whether conventional or herbal, can help to reduce both the inflammation and the irritation. Sometimes it may be necessary to take *medicines (conventional, homœopathic or herbal)* by mouth, in order to reduce the irritation and inflammation. It has been shown recently that some specific Chinese herbs taken by mouth seem to clear up completely even severe eczema in a number of people, especially children. And often a soak in a bath of lukewarm water with a handful of sodium bicarbonate in it can be very soothing, particularly if a large area of skin is itching. Bath oils, such as lavender oil, baby oil and others also have their place in the management of these chronic conditions. Cosmetic bath oils, cubes and so on, should be avoided, especially those that are scented or coloured.

The *standard AT exercises* can help to reduce the stress which may be a contributory factor, and thereby reduce the severity of the condition or even eliminate it altogether. These exercises also help to alleviate the itching, but remember that the *warmth exercises* may have to be modified or even eliminated if they increase the irritation. If that happens, substitute 'slightly cool' (in the limbs) – NEVER 'cold'.

It is well known that both eczema and psoriasis can be triggered or greatly aggravated by intense emotions, especially repressed ones. Anger and frustration seem to figure particularly prominently in these cases – and, of course, these feelings can also be caused by the condition. So you should find the *offloading exercises* (lesson 5) of immense value here. You may have to try a whole range of them before you find the one(s) that is (are) particularly helpful. You can, of course, use *positive affirmations* to control both the itching and the disease itself (lessons 9 and 10 and §42). Here are a few examples:

'My —— [affected part] is cool.'
'My —— [affected part] is free from irritation.'
'My skin is smooth and velvety.'
'My skin is free from disease.'
'My skin [or affected part] is cool and smooth.'
'My skin has no space for eczema (psoriasis, or urticaria).'

§52 Sleep disorders

Sleep is an extremely important state, during which most of the renovation and regeneration of worn-out or damaged tissues in the body, as well as the healing processes essential to the mind, take place. This state is controlled by the recuperation-orientated parasympathetic system (§1), and any long-term sleep disturbance can give rise to adverse physical, psychological or mental changes. Sound sleep is also important for the proper functioning of the unconscious, as it is while the conscious mind is asleep that the unconscious can deal with and offload, through the intervention of dreams, any unresolved feelings, emotions or memories.

Whether or not we are aware that we have dreamt, the offloading of emotions by the unconscious proceeds while we are asleep. However, it is useful to be able to record the dreams that you do remember, as soon as you wake up. The dreams themselves are not quite as important as the feelings, emotions and memories that may be associated with or triggered by your recording of them. Being aware of these feelings can be a very effective starting-point for dealing with unresolved problems.

Sleeping problems are amongst the commonest of all human experiences, and sleep can become disturbed for a number of reasons. It is important to remember, though, that the amount of sleep required by different individuals, and even the amount required by one person at different times in his or her life, can vary considerably. Some people find that they need only four or five hours' sleep, while others feel shattered and physically unwell if they have anything less than eight or nine. Furthermore, the type of disturbance also varies. Some people have great difficulty in getting off to sleep; others find that they wake in the early hours and are unable to get back to sleep; yet others find that although they can get to sleep all right they wake up several times during the night, and so feel shattered the next day. Remember that although sleep disturbances may seem to happen for no apparent reason, there is always a reason. And the reason why the cause so often eludes us is usually because, either consciously or unconsciously, we do not want to admit to its existence.

The commonest causes of a disturbed sleeping pattern are anxiety, fear, depression, pain, excessive amounts of unused energy resulting from insufficient exercise; boredom, dissatisfaction with one's achievements during the day, inability to switch off the stresses associated with work, family or other commitments; and shift work. Chronic loss or disturbance of sleep can lead to fatigue and lethargy, impaired efficiency in all tasks, and lack of concentration and attention – all of which are compounded and aggravated by sleeping tablets, tranquillisers and alcohol, if you use them in order to sleep better!

What can I do?

First of all, try to find out *why* you cannot sleep. Be honest with yourself, and if you find that the problem has to do with marital, psychological or social problems, do seek the help of a *counsellor, therapist* or *other professional. Avoid drinking stimulant or caffeine-containing drinks*, especially tea and coffee, late in the evening. (You may have to stop drinking them after 5 or 6 pm.) Try replacing such drinks with herbal teas, especially those known to be relaxing, such as camomile and comfrey. Hot milky drinks taken last thing at night can also be helpful. Contrary to popular belief, alcohol can actually interfere with sleep rather than improve it. If you have a lot of physical tension, that too may interfere with your sleeping, and a good routine of daily *exercise, professional massage* or *motor-loosening exercises* (lesson 5) can be of great help in this context.

The *standard AT exercises* offer the most effective method of getting to sleep. AUTOGENIC TRAINING IS ALSO AN EFFECTIVE WAY OF TRYING TO COME OFF SLEEPING TABLETS. However, if it is to be used for this purpose you must first learn and practise the technique thoroughly. Then you may have to reduce the dosage gradually, especially if you are heavily dependent on the sleeping tablets or have been taking them for a long time.

When you use the standard exercises to get off to sleep, your attitude and position are very important. Make sure that you are warm and comfortable, and get into your favourite sleeping position – but do not lie on your stomach, as that can make you feel uncomfortable, especially after eating. You MUST NOT do your AT thinking 'I am going to do my AT in order to fall asleep'. This attitude brings both active concentration and the 'rat' (§4) into their own, and thus interferes with the beneficial effects of AT. YOU MUST DEVELOP THE FULL PASSIVE ATTITUDE that says, 'I am going to enjoy my AT, and whether or not I fall asleep is immaterial'. With this attitude, it is bound to work.

Occasionally people find that they cannot do their AT before going to sleep, as it either wakes them up or makes them feel anxious. When that happens it often means that there is a deep fear of some sort, usually to do with loss in the broadest sense. Here AT may have triggered the fear of loss of control, loss of consciousness or even death, especially if you have had a near-death or a bad anaesthetic experience. If you become aware of this and externalise it through one of the methods mentioned in lesson 5, you will find that it helps to get rid of your problem, and you will then be able to get to sleep normally. If, on the other hand, you find that you are unable to deal with it on your own, you may require the help of a professional counsellor or therapist.

As in so many other conditions, the *offloading exercises* are very helpful in enabling you to deal with any underlying fears or emotional troubles that may be contributing towards your sleeplessness. One of the most effective for sleeping problems, especially if you have a lot of underlying muscle tension or if your limbs jump in the night, is the *motor-loosening exercise* (page 90). What you should do is have a short session with this exercise, and then go to bed and do your AT. If you happen to wake in the night and have difficulty in getting off again, get up and do the motor-loosening exercise (having first gone into another room so that you will not disturb your partner, if you have one). Then go back to bed, do your AT and go to sleep. It really does work – as confirmed by all those who have tried it! The *positive affirmations* (lessons 9 and 10) can help to enhance and reinforce the normal beneficial effects of AT. The sort of phrases that you can use are:

'I feel comfortable, cosy and sleepy.'
'Warmth makes me relaxed and sleepy.'
'I sleep easily and comfortably.'
'It sleeps me.'
'I know that I'll sleep through.'
'My sleep will be uninterrupted.'
'Sleep comes easily.'
'I am warm and comfortable and sleep comes easily.'
'Warmth makes me sleepy. It sleeps me.'
'Darkness makes me comfortable and sleepy.'
'Darkness helps me sleep easily.'

You can, of course, make up your own phrases to suit your needs and personality.

§53 Smoking

Although smoking can be just a habit for some people, others can be truly dependent on it – physically, psychologically or both. It can be very difficult for these people to give it up.

Apart from being a socially unpleasant and currently unacceptable habit in many settings and situations, smoking contributes to many of the more serious medical problems, such as heart attacks, strokes, stomach ulcers and cancers, especially lung and stomach cancer. Its detrimental effect on the lungs make it one of the major causes of chronic disability, such as bronchitis and emphysema. Anyone who has watched a victim of one of these diseases gasping for breath even at the slightest exertion, will realise how utterly miserable and wretched such conditions can be. Smoking can also lead to circulatory problems, especially in the legs, which at best cause difficulty in walking and at worst lead to gangrene and amputation. (See also §§6, 14, 17, 19, 21, 22, 23, 24, 31, 35, 43, 46, 61.)

It is therefore imperative that all smokers try to give up smoking, in order to prevent any of these disabling ailments from developing.

As stress is often one of the reasons why people resort to smoking, it is important to find out where the sources of stress or conflict lie. You may find – if stress is behind your smoking problem – that discovering its cause will make it easier for you to give up. MOTIVATION, PLUS DETERMINATION TO GIVE UP, ARE, OF COURSE, EXTREMELY IMPORTANT. You will never be able to give up if you are trying to do so just because someone else wants you to!

What can I do?

Good nutrition is important, as are *nutritional supplements*, especially vitamin C and the B group. One of the B vitamins, nicotinic acid, is known to improve circulation. *Exercise* can improve your general condition and increase the circulation of blood to the various organs and tissues which may have been partially deprived of oxygen by your inhaling smoke. Nicotine-impregnated chewing gum can sometimes be of help, but unfortunately some people can actually become addicted to that as well! So if you do use it, make sure that you plan your withdrawal properly and stick to the routine that you have chosen. If you are not careful, you can actually get addicted to both cigarettes and chewing gum! *Acupuncture* has been shown to help some smokers.

Autogenic training can help to remove background stress, which is a significant contributory factor to so many of the problems discussed in this book. Also, by centring you – that is, focusing on your inner self – AT will help you to become aware of any other aspects of your life that may need sorting out, thus enabling you to deal with them. In addition, AT helps you to get your priorities right, and that in itself will make it a lot easier for you to give up smoking anyway.

The experience of one of my own trainees will probably explain this better. Mike had come on the AT course ostensibly in order to give up smoking, as he had tried everything, and with no success. AT was going to be his last throw. Once he had completed the course, he decided to use the phrase 'Smoking gives me up' as an affirmation. When he came out of his AT state after his first attempt at using it, he said that, despite his intention, the sentence that actually came up was 'I am calm and centred'! 'Thinking about my life, it makes perfect sense, of course,' he pointed out. He had recently been made redundant, and his marriage was breaking up. He therefore decided to use the sentence that had come to him spontaneously, until the review session eight weeks later. When he returned and was asked how he had got on, he said that he had worked on his confidence as well as his other problems, and had managed to get himself a new job. He and his wife were seeing a marriage guidance counsellor, and were sorting their relationship out. Since most of the causes of stress in his life were being attended to, he had no difficulty in giving up smoking. He did not even have to resort to one of the positive affirmations that are designed for giving up smoking.

Positive affirmations (lessons 9 and 10) can, though, be of great help in reinforcing the general beneficial effects of the *standard AT exercises*, as well as in making it easier for you to give up smoking. You can try any of these, or make up your own:

'Tobacco tastes foul and revolting.'
'I have no desire to smoke.'
'Smoking is immaterial.'
'I dislike the taste and smell of tobacco (cigarettes).'
'I have no need for smoking.'
'Smoking is an unnecessary activity.'
'I don't need to smoke to calm my nerves.'
'Smoking is an antisocial habit, and therefore easy to give up.'
'Smoking revolts me.'
'Smoking gives me up.'

§54 Sport

People involved in sport these days are subject to a great many stresses, both physical and psychological; enormous demands are made of them, and their remuneration has dramatically increased. They all tend to drive themselves harder and harder, in pursuit of more and more difficult goals – indeed, goals that would have been thought impossible only a few years ago. It is partly because of all this that some sportsmen and women are resorting to drugs, not only to help them relax and cope with their lives more effectively, but also to improve their performances – as demonstrated in the 1988 Olympics.

Apart from the usual everyday stresses that, like everyone else, sportsmen are subject to, they have to cope with the kinds of stress, fear and anxiety that arise from frequent travelling (see §30); from being away from their families and friends; and from spending long periods in hotels and other strange places. Then there is the intense physical, emotional and psychological stress of the actual competition, which includes the stage fright to which a great many seem to be subject, irrespective of their sport. All this was well demonstrated by a study carried out on the Japanese Olympic competitors taking part in the 1960 Olympics in Rome.

What can I do?

The right *diet* and *nutritional supplements* are, of course, crucial aspects of the sportsman's or woman's daily life. They are to some extent dictated by his or her particular sporting activity. *Massage*, without oils or with them (*aromatherapy*), *physiotherapy*, *hydrotherapy*, *osteopathy*, *chiropractic* and *acupuncture* can be of considerable help both in preventing injuries and traumas and in healing injured parts.

Autogenic training has been used in many sports, including *golf, baseball, tennis, judo, skiing, cycling, hockey, shooting* and *football*. Many beneficial effects have been observed in ALL sportsmen and women who have used the technique regularly as a part of their training programme. It is important to appreciate, though, that THE RESULTS ARE NOT INSTAN-TANEOUS, and if you wish to gain the maximum benefit from the practice of AT you must learn the technique at least one season before any major event or competition at which you wish to excel.

It has been shown that sportspersons using the *standard exercises* have been able to control the normal stresses, anxieties and fears associated with international competition. These exercises have also been found to be of great help in centring them and keeping them calm and relaxed before their events. Occasionally, in certain individuals, the use of 'My forehead is cool and clear' can trigger an attack of anxiety or agitation. This is uncommon, but if it affects you in this way, don't use that formula. Concentration on the *warmth exercises* can be particularly effective in this case. *Imagery*, both *guided and spontaneous*, can be an extremely useful tool in your mental rehearsal and preparation. Most of the sports-men in the 1960 survey found that they could use the deep AT state to mentally rehearse their performance, thereby making it easier to cope in the actual event. This was particularly useful as they could rehearse in this way anywhere and anytime, even if they had no access to their training facilities.

The other benefits of AT as far as sport is concerned seem to be *better performance and co-ordination, better endurance* and *faster recuperation*. The improved performance seems to be due to a reduction in fear and anxiety (the stage-fright element) as well as in muscle tension. The fact that with AT you can refresh yourself and replenish your energy source repeatedly allows you to train for longer periods without getting exhausted, mentally or physically. Using this method also makes the actual training sessions pass more quickly and more enjoyably.

The *offloading exercises*, especially the *motor-* and the *noise-loosening* ones, can be particularly effective in releasing tension from specific muscle groups (pages 90–91). The *posi-tive affirmations* (lessons 9 and 10) can play a central role in improving your overall performance. They can boost confidence and assertiveness, maintain a positive, winning attitude and overcome any feelings of inferiority. They can help you to overcome any doubts that you may have about your ability not only to compete with the best but to win – especially if a giant in your particular field is intimidating you.

The *partial exercise*, 'My neck and shoulders are heavy', as well as affirmations such as 'I am calm under pressure', can help to maintain a state of calm, relaxation, co-ordination and confidence throughout a game or event. If your sport has natural breaks, as with tennis or snooker, the repeated use of a *short exercise* such as 'My right (left) arm is heavy' can be extremely useful during these breaks, both to keep you calm and confident and to enable you to refresh yourself whenever you want to, especially if you are required to perform for longer than expected, as can happen with such sports as tennis and snooker. Do remember, though, if you do this, to CANCEL ADEQUATELY, so that your performance and reflexes return to normal as as soon as you resume your game or event.

§55 Stuttering

This is a very distressing habit which is invariably aggravated by stress, tension, fear and anxiety. As there can be many underlying causes, including heredity, left-handedness, physical defects, infantile conflicts, sexual maladjustment and social fear, a number of different treatments may be adopted. These can include play or group therapy, counselling, surgical correction of any physical deformity, psycho-drama, and analytical therapy in conjunction with autogenic training.

Autogenic training has a particularly important role to play by virtue of its ability to induce a passive state of relaxation and thus remove any underlying stress that may be implicated in the stuttering. The technique can be successfully applied to anyone older than nine, and occasionally it has been taught to particularly mature six- and seven-year-olds. For young children, limit the exercises to the *heaviness*, *warmth* and *cooling* ones, and exclude the abdominal warmth, heartbeat and breathing exercises. There are a number of positive benefits for this age group, apart from improvement in speech, including a reduction in tension, anxiety and fear. Children who have undergone AT also become more sociable and friendly with playmates, parents and teachers; there is an improvement in the classroom, as well as in play activities (see also §29).

The *standard exercises* help to generally relax the adolescent or adult sufferer, considerably reducing the stress-related aspect of his or her condition. The frequent use of 'My neck and shoulders are heavy and warm', especially before and while talking, can be extremely helpful. The *offloading exercises*, especially the one that deals with anxiety, and the *motor- and noise-loosening exercises*, can be of marked value, as can *positive affirmations* such as:

'Speaking does not matter. It speaks me.'
'My speech is automatic and unimpeded.'
'I speak freely and easily.'
'I enjoy speaking. It is free and easy.'
'I am free and confident about speaking.'

§56 Thrush (Candida)

This is a relatively common infection which can present acutely, as happens in babies' mouths or a woman's vagina. It commonly follows a period of being run down or tired, or after taking antibiotics for some other infection. It can also be present in a chronic form in those who are on antibiotic treatment on a long-term basis, or whose immunity is compromised as happens in AIDS and ME.

What can I do?

It is best to see your own doctor first, to have the correct diagnosis made. There are some specific medications that your GP can give you to try to eradicate the disease. However, there are a number of things that you can do yourself to prevent the infection taking hold, or to try and get rid of it once it has become established, in conjunction with what your GP might give you.

Have a well-balanced diet with plenty of fruit and vegetables, and nutritional supplements if necessary. Avoid mushrooms or any other yeast- or sugar-containing food or drink, especially if you are already infected with thrush. Garlic has been found to be beneficial in combating thrush infection, as have olive oil and ginseng taken by mouth. Vitamin C is also quite beneficial, especially in doses of 1–3 grams a day (see §6).

When antibiotics are taken, as well as destroying the bacteria that cause the infection, they also destroy some of the essential non-disease-producing bacteria that are normally present in the body, such as *Lactobacillus acidophilus*. The space left by this destruction is usually filled by thrush. In order to try and prevent this from happening, you must have plenty of vitamin B while taking antibiotics, as well as supplementing your diet with *acidophilus*, which is present in certain forms of 'live' yoghurt. It can also be obtained in the form of capsules or powder which can be taken additionally during the day.

Autogenic training is of course useful both in building up the individual's immune system generally (§,13, 21 and 40) as well as helping him to recover from any underlying condition that may be contributing towards the onset of this infection (see §48).

§57 Thyroid overactivity

The thyroid gland, situated in the neck, is responsible for the body's metabolism. Sometimes it starts to overwork, thereby causing an increase in the body's activity rate. It is as if the body gets stuck in overdrive, and the effect is extremely distressing. The overactivity may or may not be accompanied by swelling of the thyroid gland itself. The common symptoms of thyroid overactivity (hyperthyroidism) are increased heart rate, sweating, intolerance of warm atmospheres, loss of weight, trembling, diarrhoea, irritability, and sometimes protrusion of the eyes.

What can I do?

Once the diagnosis has been made, the condition can be treated with medications, radioactive-iodine, surgery, or a combination of two or more of these. It has been shown that *standard autogenic training exercises* over a period of two to four months can alleviate all the symptoms, even in the absence of conventional treatment, provided that they are practised regularly. However, AT does not seem to be particularly effective if the thyroid gland is nodular and enlarged, or if there is evidence of cancer. **It is important to consult your GP and, as advised throughout this book, to use your AT in conjunction with any other treatments that may be recommended.** *Offloading exercises* and *positive affirmations* can, of course, be used to help to control specific symptoms (lessons 5, 9 and 10).

§58 Thyroid underactivity

In this condition, the symptoms are the reverse of those that characterise thyroid overactivity: that is, the individual gains weight, feels tired and lethargic and has a slow pulse; occasionally he or she experiences swelling of the ankles and lower legs, loss of hair, hoarse voice; he or she may feel cold, and may suffer from constipation, puffy eyelids, and menstrual disturbances in the case of women. Underactive thyroid (hypothyroidism, or myxoedema) is usually treated with tablets to replace the naturally occurring hormone which, in this condition, the body is failing to produce in sufficient amounts. Treatment is usually lifelong. Sufficient amounts of iodine, obtained from food and water, are essential for the proper functioning of the thyroid gland. The foods that are rich in iodine are kelp, vegetables grown in iodine-rich soil, onions and all seafoods. If you are suffering from thyroid disease and think that you may need extra iodine, it is best to consult your GP or nutritionist first, for his or her advice.

What can I do?

It has been shown that a moderate degree of thyroid underactivity can be corrected by the regular use of *autogenic training*, **in conjunction with replacement therapy**. AT's apparent ability to normalise the functioning of the thyroid gland is believed to be due to the natural regulating and healing processes that are triggered by the regular practice of the technique. Do make sure that you use all aspects of autogenic training, to obtain maximum benefit in this condition.

§59 Torticollis

This is an uncommon, and very distressing, condition. It is characterised by intermittent spasm of the large muscles on one side of the neck, producing a sudden and painful turning of the neck to that side. Occasionally the spasm becomes permanent. If this occurs, it is best for the sufferer to be fully assessed, to ensure that there is no serious underlying physical condition needing specific treatment.

What can I do?

Once it has been confirmed that there are no serious underlying causes, you can help yourself in a number of ways. Conventional medical treatment is very inadequate, though a few people are helped by certain drugs. *Herbal or homœopathic medicines* which relieve muscle spasm can be helpful, as can *reflexology, massage, osteopathy, chiropractic, physiotherapy* and *spiritual healing*.

Autogenic training helps greatly by reducing tension and spasm in the affected muscles, thus enabling them to relax properly and helping you to overcome the problem. If there is a strong emotional element, as there can be with any muscular problem, the *offloading exercises* (lesson 5) can be very effective. And *positive affirmations* (lessons 9 and 10) can work on the actual area. Try:

'My neck and shoulders are heavy and warm.'
'The spasm is immaterial; it relaxes.'
'My neck muscles are free and easy.'
'My neck muscles are relaxed and comfortable.'
'No tension or spasm exists in my neck muscles.'
'I am free of neck muscle spasm.'

There are many others that you can make up yourself, or see §§16, 18, 31, 39, 42 and 44.

§60 Tranquilliser habituation (addiction)

With the development of the more sophisticated tranquillisers, particularly the benzodiazipine group, we thought that
we had found a panacea for the management of nervous
disorders such as anxiety and sleeplessness. It was believed
originally that they had no long-term side effects, and only
caused a possible temporary drowsiness and slowing of the
reflexes in a few people. Unfortunately, it has only recently
been discovered that if you take these drugs for more than two
to four weeks, habituation as well as true addiction can occur.
Habituation means that the individual takes the drugs purely
as a habit and, if he stops taking them, suffers no physical
withdrawal symptoms. However, true addiction means that
the sufferer becomes physically dependent on the drug and
develops mild to severe physical withdrawal symptoms, such
as exacerbation of anxiety symptoms, palpitations, sweating
and extreme irritability and restlessness, if the drug is stopped
even slowly.

Side effects can include an exacerbation of depression and
the onset of rage reactions. On withdrawal there can be
severe symptoms akin to the original anxiety, including sleep
disturbances, but even worse than the original condition for
which they were prescribed. It can take up to six months to
work through the withdrawal symptoms. The problem is
compounded because not only may you have to deal with
these symptoms, but you also have to face up to the unresolved problems which were left in abeyance when you first
began to take the drug. To have to deal with both problems
simultaneously can be quite a daunting prospect.

We must, of course, appreciate that some people's problems are too distressing or insoluble for them to cope with
without the help of tranquillisers: despite advice to the contrary they may decide to go on taking them, seeing this as the
least of the evils available to them. We must respect this

choice, since, as I have already mentioned, the eventual decision as regards what to do with himself and his life has to be the individual's alone, provided that he is fully aware of the disadvantages, as well as the advantages, of his chosen course. We should not forget that some people need to take drugs of this kind for specific conditions such as epilepsy and muscle spasm; for these people it could be quite dangerous to discontinue their drugs, especially suddenly and without the supervision of a doctor. So if you are intending to come off tranquillisers, discuss your intention with your doctor, as you may require close supervision and support when you embark on such a venture. The dosage will usually need to be reduced very gradually.

Tranquillisers did seem to be the easy way out for both doctor and patient, as they were quickly dispensed and quickly taken, and in this instant-results society the collusion appeared to satisfy both parties. But by adopting this attitude all we did was deny and repress the real causes of our problems, and rather than work hard to deal with them we allowed them to lie hidden, at least from our conscious selves, behind a convenient veil of drug-induced denial.

What can I do?

The most important thing is, of course, PREVENTION – so that you never find yourself in such dire straits that you need to resort to tranquillisers or sleeping tablets in order to obliterate, albeit superficially, your problems. FOR YOU MUST NOT FORGET THAT THE UNRESOLVED DIFFICULTY WILL REMAIN STORED IN THE UNCONSCIOUS AND CONTINUE TO TROUBLE YOU UNTIL YOU RESOLVE IT.

If you have been on tranquillisers for some time and feel that you are habituated or addicted to them, there are things that you can do to help yourself come off them and at the same time minimise the withdrawal reactions. TRY TO CUT DOWN ON CAFFEINE-CONTAINING AND OTHER STIMULANT DRINKS, as they can exacerbate symptoms such as palpitations and trembling. *Drink calming herbal teas* instead, such as camomile, comfrey and fennel. Hot milky drinks, especially last thing at night, can be quite helpful. You can also try *herbal or homœopathic compounds*, as well as therapeutic methods such as *massage* –

especially if you have a lot of muscular tension – *reflexology* or *acupuncture*. The help of *a good friend who will listen to you and support you*, or *a professional counsellor or therapist*, can be invaluable, as they can help you to cope not only with your withdrawal symptoms but also with any of the unresolved emotions, feelings, memories or problems that drove you to use tranquillisers in the first place. *Self-support groups* can also be a great help in enabling you to kick the habit (see Appendix).

The *standard AT exercises* can, of course, be of great benefit here, whether in preventing you from going on to sedatives and tranquillisers or in helping you to come off them. As a preventive measure they enable you to deal with the stresses of everyday life, and if you are already on tranquillisers you can use the exercises to reduce background stress – or at least make it much more manageable for yourself. When that happens, you will find that your need for tranquillisers will diminish, and you will be able gradually to cut down your dosage. Do remember to reduce the dosage slowly, so that any withdrawal effects can be minimised. You will find that, to cope with withdrawal symptoms, you can use the sentence 'My neck and shoulders are heavy and warm' to great benefit, by frequently repeating it between your regular full exercises (lesson 2). To top up your feeling of relaxation and peace, the *short exercise*, 'My right (left) arm is heavy', can be immensely helpful (lesson 1).

Again, the *offloading exercises* are invaluable in permitting you to deal with any unresolved feelings or emotions that you may be harbouring. The *motor-loosening exercise* can help to deal with excessive muscle tension (lesson 5). You can, of course, use the *positive affirmations* in order to enhance the general effects of AT, as well as to control unpleasant withdrawal symptoms (lessons 9 and 10). The sentences that can be used include:

'I am calm and content.'
'I feel safe and secure without the tranquillisers.'
'I know that I can do it if I try.'
'I can give up —— [name the tranquilliser] easily and without problems.'
'—— [name the tranquilliser] is unnecessary.'

'I am happier and more content without —— [name the tranquilliser].'

'My body and mind can do without —— [name the tranquilliser].'

'I feel much better without —— [name the tranquilliser].'

As usual, you can use other phrases to suit your personality or, in this case, your particular withdrawal symptom(s).

Those who have come off tranquillisers with autogenic training have usually found that they needed to use all its aspects for maximum benefit, especially during the initial withdrawal phase.

§61   Ulcers, indigestion and hiatus hernia

'Indigestion' is the common factor connecting stomach inflammation (gastritis), stomach and duodenal ulcer and hiatus hernia, and that is the reason why they are all included in this section. 'Ulcer' in this context refers to the appearance of a break in the superficial layers of the stomach or duodenum (upper part of the small bowel), and can occur at any age. It may be caused by a number of factors – smoking, drinking excessive amounts of coffee or alcohol, intake of unsuitable foods, such as when it is of poor quality or too spicy. The most important factor, of course, is stress. Hiatus hernia is a condition in which the muscles of the lower part of the gullet and the upper part of the stomach become weakened, allowing the stomach acids to reach these delicate areas with the ensuing symptoms of indigestion or heartburn.

Pain is another common symptom which, together with a feeling of indigestion, appears in the upper abdomen and lower chest; it is usually intermittent and associated with food, either before or after meals. A bloated feeling, or heartburn with occasional nausea and vomiting, are also quite common. These conditions may also be associated with loss of appetite. Sometimes the pain or discomfort occurs in the early hours of the morning and wakes the sufferer up. This usually happens if acid stomach contents rise up into the lower part of the gullet, which is not designed to withstand them. The symptoms are triggered or aggravated by fried and other fatty food, as well as hot and spicy food, alcohol, coffee and strong tea; by infection; by smoking; and most important of all, by STRESS, including that associated with repressed or unresolved emotions such as anxiety and anger. This last was recognised by traditional medical practitioners even before the current awareness of stress as a contributory factor to many serious diseases.

If indigestion persists for longer than two weeks, and

especially if you have never had it before, you must consult your GP. Whatever the cause, there is a lot that you can do to try and prevent it from occurring in the first place and alleviating it once it has developed.

What can I do?

The most important thing, as implied above, is to PREVENT INDIGESTION FROM OCCURRING BY AVOIDING THE FOODS THAT CAUSE IT. Also, *avoid alcoholic drinks* (especially in excess), *smoking, coffee and strong tea*, as well as chemicals that are known to cause trouble, such as aspirin; and, finally, TRY TO DEAL WITH ANY STRESS OR REPRESSED EMOTIONS.

Once you develop the symptoms, on a regular basis, it is best to consult your GP to exclude any possible serious underlying causes. That done, there is still a lot you can do to help alleviate your symptoms. During the acute phase it may be worthwhile resting both yourself and your stomach by having *frequent light meals* such as grilled or boiled chicken or fish, with boiled or steamed white rice. *Avoid raw fruit and vegetables*, although they can be eaten, lightly boiled or steamed, in moderate amounts. Try to stick to *herbal teas*, especially those known to be relaxing, such as camomile and comfrey. Slippery elm has been found to be very beneficial in lining the gullet and the stomach and thus improving the symptoms dramatically. If you can tolerate milk, have *plenty of milky drinks* as well, but do remember that if you are allergic to ordinary milk its use can exacerbate your symptoms. Make sure that you take plenty of *nutritional supplements* (§§ 5 and 6), especially vitamin C, which is known to help with healing wounds and ulcers — but do make sure that you take in in the buffered soluble form. This means that the solution of vitamin C, which is normally acidic, has been manufactured in such a way that it is *neutral* and therefore does not aggravate the symptoms.

If you find that you are getting pain or indigestion at night, use several pillows, so that you are semi-propped up while you sleep. *Standard antacids* can be of great help, as can *homœopathic and herbal medicines*. Also, antispasmodics can reduce spasm in the muscles of the stomach and bowel wall, thus helping to reduce the pain as well as to promote healing.

There are medicines now available that can reduce the production of stomach acids, which are thought to be one of the main physiological causes of the condition, as well as other medicines that help to heal ulcers. These can only be prescribed by your doctor. **And do consult your doctor** for a proper diagnosis of the cause of your symptoms if they do not settle down quickly when you have tried all the treatments I have just described.

Autogenic training plays a particularly important role in the management of indigestion, ulcers and hiatus hernia:

1   AT helps to reduce the general level of stress, thereby reducing the acid secretions of the stomach.
2   It reduces muscle spasm in the walls of the stomach and bowel, and by regulating the bowel's movements it promotes good digestion as well as the speedy passage of food from the stomach to the bowel, so that there is no stagnation in the stomach, which can lead to flatulence, feelings of bloatedness or nausea.
3   The *offloading exercises* enable you to deal with any repressed emotions that may be contributing to your symptoms.
4   *Positive affirmations* can further alleviate your symptoms. For instance the use of the sentence, 'My stomach is cool (warm, heavy)' – depending on what feels right – can be of great benefit in reducing pain and discomfort.

If you suffer from any of these conditions you should practise the exercise 'My solar plexus is warm' with some care, as in a few trainees the pain can at first actually get worse. If it does, leave this sentence out altogether, and perhaps reintroduce it once you have relaxed sufficiently and consequently alleviated the symptoms. As most trainees seem to benefit from this particular sentence, you will just have to try it and see how it feels. But be sensible and gentle with yourself, and if you find that you do get untoward feelings, then leave it out. Doing so will not reduce the effectiveness of your AT in the long run (see also lesson 7).

§62 Urinary problems

In considering urinary symptoms such as excessive frequency, pain when urinating, urine retention and having to get up in the night, we have to distinguish between those that have some psychological origin and those that are associated with an underlying physical condition such as an infection, a mechanical obstruction or a tumour. If you suffer from any persistent urinary problem, **do have it investigated straight away** so that you can find out what the underlying cause is. Regular drinking of one or two glasses of cranberry juice daily can be very effective in preventing attacks of cystitis as well as helping to relieve the symptoms during acute attacks. Once that has been established, you can use AT to great benefit.

It has been found that in most people with psychogenic urinary symptoms, such as excessive frequency when they are nervous, inability to pass urine in a public place, or habitually needing to get up during the night, *autogenic training exercises* seem to alleviate or clear the symptoms completely. If there are any residual symptoms, *positive affirmations* (lessons 9 and 10) are very useful. Try these:

'My bladder is warm (heavy).'
'It empties when it is full.'
'I don't need to go so frequently.'
'I will only urinate when my bladder is full.'
'My bladder has no spasm.'
'I have a good stream.'
'My urine flows freely and comfortably.'

You can make up other phrases to suit your situation or personality, as outlined in lessons 9 and 10 and for the relief of pain see §42.

APPENDICES

Appendix 1 Complementary therapies

Brief descriptions of various therapies, and the main centres and associations from which further information can be obtained. All the organisations listed will be happy to provide further information, including reading material.

If you decide to use any form of complementary therapy, it is very important to make sure that the practitioner is properly qualified to offer the service or treatment that you require. It is therefore advisable to check his or her credentials with the society or organisation with whom the practitioner is registered. The list that follows is by no means complete, and if the particular organisation is not mentioned here, it does not mean that it is not a bona fide organisation. It is best to check it with the British Complementary Medicine Association (BCMA), 249 Fosse Road South, Leicester LE3 1AE. (0116 2825511), or with the British Holistic Medical Association, 59 Lansdowne Place, Hove, East Sussex BN3 1FL. (01273 725951).

Acupuncture The ancient Chinese system of using needles to prevent and treat illness, by influencing the body's energy patterns.

British Acupuncture Council, Park House, 206 Latimer Road, London W10 6RE.   (0181 964 0222).
British Medical Acupuncture Society, Newton House, Newton Lane, Whitley, Warrington, Cheshire WA4 4JA. (0192 5730727)

Alexander technique A gentle technique affecting well-being by changing the individual's posture and movement. Mainly used for postural difficulties.

Society of Teachers of the Alexander Technique, 20 London House, 266 Fulham Road, London SW10 9EL. (0171-351 0828)

Aromatherapy   A wide-ranging system of massage using natural oils for specific purposes. Used where progress is required through body-based work.

International Federation of Aromatherapists, Stamford
   House, 2-4 Chiswick High Road, London W4 1TH.
   (0181-742 2605).
Aromatherapy Organisations Council, PO Box 355,
   Croydon CR9 2QP.   (0181-251 7912).
Register of Qualified Aromatherapists, PO Box 3431,
   Danbury, Chelmsford, Essex CM3 4UA.   (01245
   227957)

Art therapy   Employs drawing, painting, pattern-making and other art techniques to resolve blocks and problems and to promote well-being. Used where a person wants to explore more fully the potential for change.

British Association of Art Therapists, 11a Richmond Road,
   Brighton, Sussex BN2 3RL.

Autogenic training   A simple but effective method of relaxation, enabling the body, the mind and the emotions to get in touch with each other and to start functioning in harmony, thus enabling the individual to feel whole and complete.

British Association for Autogenic Training (BAFATT),
   c/o Royal Homœopathic Hospital, Great Ormond Street,
   London WC1N 3HR (please send SAE).
Dr Kai Kermani BSc. MBBS, LRCP, MRCS, DRCOG
   MRCGP MBFATT, Holistic Health, Healing and Auto-
   genic Centre, 10 Connaught Hill, Loughton, Essex
   IG10 4DU.

Bach flower remedies   These are all prepared from flowers of wild plants, bushes and trees, and none of them are harmful or addictive. They are mainly used to affect the individual's mood and state of mind, as it is known that fear, apprehension and worry often interfere with the body's proper healing processes.

Dr Edward Bach Centre, Mount Vernon, Sotwell, Walling-
   ford, Oxfordshire OX10 0PZ.   (01491 839489)

Breathing therapy A range of approaches that focus on breathing to ease distress and promote well-being: for instance, 'rebirthing', which emphasises the individual's release from the birth trauma. Particularly useful where there are difficulties with breathing and where progress through body-based work is required.

Chiropractic Focuses on skeletal malfunctioning, particularly spinal problems; treatment is by manipulation. Useful for problems to do with muscles, bones and joints.

British Chiropractic Association, Bragrave House, 17 Bragrave Street, Reading RG1 1QB. (0118 9505950).

Conventional (orthodox) therapy refers to the usual method of treatment adopted by most doctors. This basically includes chemotherapy (medications), radiotherapy and surgery.

Counselling A range of approaches (including neurolinguistic programming) that use language and communication as the principal means of effecting change. Useful where the individual wishes to tackle issues, and thereby hasten change, via dialogue. This is also a useful therapy to adopt if wishing to alter or improve interpersonal relationships, such as problems arising in marriages.

Co-counselling is a form of counselling which takes place in pairs, both the participants acting as counsellors in turn. However, unlike counselling where some form of advice is usually offered to the patient or the client, in co-counselling no advice is given by the one acting as the therapist. All that the counsellor does in this context is provide a safe and loving space and listen to his partner ('client'). It is up to the client to think of solutions once he has verbalised whatever may be worrying him. Neither of the parties need be a qualified counsellor, but both would have to have gone through a formal co-counselling training period.

British Association for Counselling, 1 Regent Place, Rugby, Warwickshire CV21 2PJ. (01788 578328)
Relate, Herbert Gray College, Little Church Street, Rugby, Warwickshire CV21 3AP. (01788 573241)

Human Potential Research Project [mainly co-counselling],
 Dept. of Educational Studies, University of Surrey, Guild-
 ford, Surrey GU2 5XH.   (01483 300800)
Westminster Pastoral Foundation [counselling training], 23
 Kensington Square, London W8 5HN.   (0171-937 6956)

Cranial osteopathy   This is a specialised form of
osteopathy in which the therapist looks for the subtle and
fine involuntary movements of the client, including the
head, and by gentle manipulation tries to balance them and
thus return the client to better health and healing.
Christian Sullivan, 6 Market Street, Bradford-on-Avon,
 Wiltshire BA15 1LH.   (01225 868282)

Dance therapy   Uses rhythmic movememnt to relieve distress and muscular tension and to improve health and well-
being. Particularly useful where the individual wishes to
accelerate change through movement, music and rhythm.
 Apart from the usual forms of dancing such as ballet,
modern, 'popular', tap and so on, there are some other
special forms that are mainly used to induce a state of physical
and mental relaxation. These include circle, meditative and
sacred, and creative dancing.
 Circle dancing is a form of dance in which the participants
dance in a circle, using different set and prearranged steps. It
can also be combined with chanting. Meditative and sacred
dancing are quite similar to circle dancing, but the specific
moves that are used go back to the sacred dances of ancient
civilisations such as the Sufis, Egyptian, Chinese or Indian.
Creative movement or dance refers to the spontaneous and
free movement of the body in response to music. This means
allowing the body to move freely as and how it wants without
inhibitory control from the conscious mind.

Circle and Sacred Dancing, c/o Rosemary Cartwright, Gaia
 Natural Therapies, London Road, Forest Row, East
 Sussex RH18 5EZ.   (01342 822716)

Death (living with dying)   A series of workshops designed to
enable those facing the prospects of fatal diseases and those
caring for them to address some of the issues raised by the
subject.

Christiann Heal, 9 Cannon Row, London NW3 1EH. (0171-435 5432)

Dietary therapy See *Nutritional therapy*

Drama therapy (psycho-drama) This is run by a qualified therapist and is in a group setting. The participants are intended to work through unresolved blocks, emotions and past traumas, by acting out the scene. Each person uses the props provided, as well as other participants in the group, as the people involved in the particular scene that the individual wants to re-enact.

British Psychodrama Association, Heather Cottage, The Clachan, Roseneath, Helensburgh, Argyle Bute, Scotland G84 0RF. (01436 831838).

Education Apart from conventional forms of education the organisation for accelerated learning uses the holistic concept of the body, mind and spirit as well as stimulation of all the senses in order to maximise both the speed and the learning abilities of students.

SEAL, PO Box 2246, Bath BA1 2YR. (01225 466244).

Exercise The use of physical movement to keep fit as well as improve the physiological state of the body.

Keep Fit Association, Francis House, Francis Street, London SW1P 1DE. (0171-233 8898)

Flower therapy Employs flower essences to improve general condition, particularly in cases of persistent ill health; also used for specific diseases. The best known flower therapy is the thirty-eight *Bach remedies* (see above). There are now a number of flower essences from other parts of the world which claim to be as effective as those of the UK.

Fun, creativity and transformational healing workshops Recovery from illness and healing in its broadest holistic sense can only occur if and when we are ready to let go of old and often negative patterns and move on to new and more positive patterns of thought and behaviour. This is the process that I call transformational healing. These workshops are designed to help the participants work through some of the negative aspects of their thought and behaviour patterns and enhance their positive attributes in a friendly, loving and supportive atmosphere. A whole range of different techniques is used. These include pictures, drawings, puppets, games, clay, masks, music, dance, relaxation, visualisation and guided imagery. Participants need not know anything about any of these techniques and everyone, especially those with catastrophic illness, is welcome.

Dr Kai Kermani, Holistic Health and Healing Centre, 10 Connaught Hill, Loughton, Essex IG10 4DU.

Healing   A range of approaches that rely upon the communication of energy, often via the hands. Useful where the individual wants to restore or strengthen his or her own healing powers.   (See also *Spiritual healing*, p. 298)

Sufi Healing Order of Great Britain, 10 Beauchamp Avenue, Leamington Spa, Warwickshire.   (Apply in writing)

Herbalism   Uses plants and plant extracts to treat both specific and general illnesses.

National Institute of Medical Herbalists, 56 Longbrook Street, Exeter, Devon EX4 6AH.   (01392 426022).
Neal's Yard Remedies, 15 Neal's Yard, Covent Garden, London WC2H 9DP.   (0171-379 7222). (Advice and a large selection of natural, herbal and homoeopathic remedies available across the counter or by post.)

Homœopathy   Uses remedies prepared from naturally occurring substances to treat the whole person, by stimulating the natural tendency of the body to heal itself.

British Homœopathic Association, 27a Devonshire Street, London W1N 1RJ   (0171-935 2163)
Register and Council of Homœopathy, 243 The Broadway, Southall, Middlesex UB1 1NF.   (0181-574 4281)
Society of Homœopaths, 2 Artisan Road, Northampton NN1 4HU.   (01604 621400).

Hydrotherapy   A technique using exercises which are performed under water, particularly helpful in situations where the affected muscles or joints are painful and stiff. Water supports and eases the discomfort of the affected areas. This form of therapy can be arranged through your local physiotherapy department, and therefore you will have to consult your own GP about it.

Hypnosis   A technique in which the patient is put in a trance of varying depths, the depth depending on the therapist and the participant. It helps to relax the individual as well as deal with some deeper unresolved conflicts (provided that the hypnotherapist is sufficiently qualified). Some individuals can be taught the art of self-hypnosis in order to try and relax when they are on their own.

British Society of Medical and Dental Hypnosis (list of medically qualified practitioners), c/o Mrs M. Samuels, 42 Links Road, Ashstead, Surrey KT21 2HJ.   (Apply by post)
Association of Hypnotists and Psychotherapists, 12 Cross Street, Nelson, Lancashire BB9 7EN.   (01282 699378)
British Hypnotherapy Association, 67 Upper Berkeley Street, London W1H 7DH.   (0171-723 4443)

Iridology   A method used for diagnosing various conditions and deficiencies, using the pupil and the back of the eye.

Guild of Naturopathic Iridologists, c/o Holistic Health College, 94 Grosvenor Road, London SW1V 3LF. (0171-834 3579)

Massage   A hands-on technique directed primarily towards the release of tension from the muscles. Particularly useful for those who wish to benefit from direct body contact.

London and Counties Society of Physiologists (for remedial massage therapists), 330 Lytham Road, Blackpool, Lancashire EY4 1DW.   (01253 408443).
Clare Maxwell-Hudson School of Massage, PO Box 457, London NW2 4BR.   (0181-450 6494)

Meditation   Covers a range of approaches used to promote a prolonged state of calm attention and awareness, for those who wish to deepen the AT state.

Transcendental Meditation, National Office, Freepost,
London SW1P 4YY.   (0990 143733)
School of Meditation (Indian method), 158 Holland Park
Avenue, London W11 4UH.   (0171-603 6116)

Music therapy   Uses music to promote a state of well-being.

British Society for Music Therapy, 69 Avondale Avenue,
East Barnet, Herts. EN4 8NB.   (0181-368 8879)
British Society for Music Therapy, Guildhall School of Music
and Drama, Barbican, London EC2Y 8DT.   (0181-368
8879)

Naturopathy Emphasises natural cures and uses such
therapies as restricted diet, manipulation, hydrotherapy,
remedial exercises and counselling.

British Register of Naturopaths, 328 Harrogate Road,
Leeds LS17 6PE.   (0113 2685992)

Nutritional therapy (dietary) Focuses on improving the
body's condition via good eating habits, vitamins and supplements.

Institute of Optimum Nutrition, 13 Blades Court, Deodar
Road, London SW15 2NU.   (0181-877 9993)
Society for Promotion of Nutritional Therapy, PO Box 47,
Heathfield, East Sussex TN21 8ZX.   (01825 872921)
Vegetarian Society UK, Parkdale, Dunham Road, Altrin-
cham, Cheshire WA14 4QG.   (0161-928 0793)

Osteopathy Focuses on musculoskeletal malfunctioning,
particularly of the spine. Massage and manipulation are used
to improve condition of muscles, joints and bones.

Osteopathic Association, 8 Boston Place, London NW1 6QH.
(0171-262 1128)

Patients' Association   An organisation that gives advice and
guidance on all aspects of patient care.

Patients' Association, PO Box 935, Harrow, Middlesex
   HA1 3YJ.   (Admin. office 0181-423 9333. Helpline
   0181-423 8999)

Polarity therapy   Concerned with promoting the free movement of energy within the body, using a range of approaches
including direct body work.

UK Polarity Association, Monomark House, 21 Old
   Gloucester Street, London WC1N 3XX.   (01886
   884121)

Psychotherapy   A broad term that incorporates any kind of
mental or emotional therapy that the individual may use, with
the aid of a qualified therapist, to help him to work through
any deep psychological problems, either individually or in
small groups. Includes analytical therapy, Gestalt, transactional therapy and psychosynthesis. Analytical psychotherapy, originally devised by Freud, is probably one of the
best known and oldest forms. It usually tends to go on for
prolonged periods as the individual gently and gradually
works through his or her past unresolved memories, emotions
and traumas by talking about them to a therapist who may
interpret the events. Gestalt is a gentle and progressive
therapy which, unlike the analytical form, concentrates on
'here and now'. Psychosynthesis and transactional therapy
are rather similar in approach: in both, the approach is
tailored to suit each individual's personality rather than the
problem.
   Too many organisations to list here, but here are just a few:

British Association of Psychotherapists, 37 Mapesbury Road,
   London NW2 4HJ.   (0181-452 9823)
British Association for Counselling, 1 Regent Place, Rugby,
   Warwickshire CV21 2PJ.   (01788 578328/9)
British Psycho-Analytical Society, 63 New Cavendish Street,
   London W1M 7RD.   (0171-580 4952)
London Centre for Psychotherapy, 32 Leighton, Kentish
   Town, London NW5 2QE.   (0171-482 2002)
Gestalt Therapy, The Gestalt Centre, 62 Paul Street,
   London EC2A 4NA.   (0171-613 4480)
Institute of Transactional Analysis, 66 Paines Lane, Pinner,
   Middlesex HA5 5BL.   (0181-866 4288)

Psychosynthesis Vision in Practice, 8 Chatsworth Road,
    London NW2 4BN.   (0171-451 2165)

Reflexology   A kind of foot massage directed towards stimulating the body's own healing processes. Used for the treatment of both specific conditions and general feelings of
unwellness.

Reflexologists' Society, c/o BCMA, 249 Fosse Road South,
    Leicester LE3 1AE.   (01242 512601)
Association of Reflexologists, Katepwa House, Ashfield
    Park, Ross-on-Wye, Hereford HR9 5AX.   (01989
    567667)

Shiatsu   A broad-based approach to massage, directed towards correcting the body's energy flow, through body-
contact therapy.

Shiatsu Society, Barber House, Fengate, Peterborough
    PE1 5YS.   (01733 758341)

Spiritual healing   A technique in which the healing energy
which is believed to be present universally is channelled
through the healer into the sufferer, to stimulate his own
inner healing powers. Can be done with or without touching
the sufferer, depending on his and the healer's wishes.

Confederation of Healing Organisations, Suite J, 2nd Floor,
    The Red-White House, 113 High Street, Berkhamsted,
    Herts. HP4 2BJ.   (01442 870660)
National Federation of Spiritual Healers, Old Manor Farm
    Studio, Church Street, Sunbury-on-Thames, Middlesex
    TW16 6RG.   (01932 783164/5)

T'ai chi   A gentle physical training enabling the individual to
use his energy, strength and power more positively.

British T'ai Chi Association, 7 Upper Wimpole Street,
    London W1.   (0171-935 8444)

Yoga   An ancient system of body postures, breath control
and meditative practices, promoting total well-being.

British Wheel of Yoga, 1 Hamilton Place, Boston Road, Sleaford, Lincs. NG34 7ES. (01529 306851)

Zoroastrianism   An ancient religion and philosophy of life based on the teachings of Zarathushtra, which believes in holism at every level of mineral, plant and animal kingdoms (including mankind).

The Zoroastrian Trust Funds of Europe, Zoroastrian House, 88 Compayne Gardens, London NW6 3RH. (0171-328 6018)

Appendix 2 Useful self-help groups and organisations

All these organisations will provide further information, including reading material. The majority would appreciate a large SAE if you apply by post.

AIDS
Terence Higgins Trust and Frontliners, 52–4 Gray's Inn Road, London WC1X 8JU. (0171-831 0330. Helpline: 0171-833 2971)
Body Positive Centre (for people who are HIV positive), 14 Greek Street, London W1V 5LE. (0171-287 8010)
AIDS Video Project, c/o Fay Kelly, PO Box 702, SW20 8SA. (Suppliers of a video, *AIDS: First steps to maximise immunity*, in which Dr Kai Kermani explains autogenic training and demonstrates the basic standard exercises and the offloading exercises. The video won the BMA Award in 1990.)

Amputated limb
British Amputee Sports Association, Harvey Rod, Aylesbury, Buck. HP21 9PP.

Anxiety
MIND (National Association for Mental Health), Granta House, 15–19 Broadway, Stratford, London E15 4BQ. (0181-519 2122)
Phobic Society, 407 Wilbraham Road, Chorlton, Manchester M21 0UT. (0161-881 1937)
Phobic Trust, 25a The Grove, Coulsdon, Surrey CR3 2BH. (0181-660 0332)
Phobic Action, Claybury Grounds, Manor Road, Woodford Green, Essex IG8 8PR. (0181-559 2551)

Arthritis
Arthritis and Rheumatism Council for Research, PO Box 177, Chesterfield, Derbyshire S4 17TQ. (01246 558033)
Arthritis Care [all forms of help and support], 18 Stephenson Way, London NW1 2HD. (0171-916 1500)

Asthma
National Asthma Campaign, Providence House, Providence Place, London N1 0NT. (0171-226 2260)

Backache
National Back Pain Association, 16 Elm Tree Road, Teddington, Middx. TW11 8ST. (0181-977 5474)

Cancer
Bristol Cancer Help Centre [for holistic approaches], Grove House, Cornwallis Grove, Clifton, Bristol BS8 4PG. (0117 9809500)
British Association of Cancer-United Patients [for information], 3 Bath Place, Rivington Street, London EC2A 3JR. (0171-613 2121)
CancerLink [contact with small groups], 11-21 Northdown Street, London N1 9BN. (0800 132905)
Cancer Relief Macmillan Fund, Anchor House, 15–19 Britten Street, London SW3 3TZ. (0171-351 7811)

Circulation
Raynaud's and Scleroderma Association, 112 Crewe Road, Alsager, Cheshire ST7 2JA. (01270 872776)

Colitis
National Association for Colitis and Crohn's Disease, 98a London Road, St Alban's, Herts. AL1 1NX. (Apply in writing)

Cystitis (see *Thrush*)

Depression
Depressives' Association, PO Box 5, Castletown, Portland, Dorset DT5 1BQ.

Manic Depression Fellowship, 8–10 High Street, Kingston-upon-Thames, Surrey KT1 1EY.   (0181 974 6550)

Heart disease
National Forum for Coronary Heart Disease Prevention, Tavistock House South, Tavistock Square, London WC1H 9LG.   (0171-383 7638)

Herpes
Herpes Virus Association (HVA), 41 North Road, London N7 9DP.   (0171-609 9061)

Migraine
Migraine Trust, 45 Great Ormond Street, London WC1N 3HZ.   (0171-831 4818)

Multiple sclerosis
Multiple Sclerosis Society of Great Britain & Northern Ireland, 25 Effie Road, London SW6 1EE.   (0171-610 7171)

Myalgic encephalomyelitis (ME)
ME Association, 4 Corringham Road, Stanford-le-Hope, Essex SS17 0AH.   (01375 642466 9am-5pm, Mon-Fri)

Obesity
Weight Watchers, Kidwells Park House, Kidwells Park Drive, Maidenhead, Berkshire SL6 8YT.   (01628 777077)
British Dietetic Association, 7th Floor, Elizabeth House, 22 Suffolk Street, Queensway, Birmingham B1 1LS. (0121-643 5483)

Parkinson's disease
Parkinson's Disease Society, 215 Vauxhall Bridge Road, London SW1V 1EJ.   (0171-931 8080)

Patients
Patients' Association, PO Box 935, Harrow, Middlesex HA1 3YJ.   (0181-423 9333)

Phobias (see *Anxiety*)

Pregnancy
British Pregnancy Advisory Service, Austy Manor, Wootton
  Wawen, Solihull B95 6DX.   (01564 793225)
Maternity Alliance, 45 Beech Street, London EC2P 2LX.
  (0171-588 8582)
National Childbirth Trust, Alexandra House, Oldham Ter-
  race, London W3 6NH.   (0181-992 8637)

Pre-menstrual syndrome and Post-natal depression
National Association for Premenstrual Syndrome, 7 Swists
  Court, High Street, Seal, Sevenoaks, Kent TN15 0EG.
  (01732 760012)

Skin ailments
National Eczema Society, 163 Eversholt Street, London
  NW1 1BU.   (0171-388 4097)
Psoriasis Association, 7 Milton Street, Northampton NN2
  7JG   (01604 711129)

Stammering
Association for Stammerers, 15 Old Ford Road, London
  E2 9PJ.   (0181-981 8818)

Stroke
The Stroke Association, Stroke House, Whitecross Street,
  London EC1.   (0171-490 7999)

Thrush
Cystitis and Candida Association, 75 Mortimer Road,
  London N1 5AR.   (0171-249 8664)

Thyroid
Hypothyroidism Self Help, 47 Crawford Avenue, Tyldesley,
  Manchester M29 8ET.   (01942 874740)

Tranquilliser addiction
CITA (Council for Involuntary Tranquilliser Addiction),
  Cavendish House, Brighton Road, Waterloo, Liverpool
  L22 5NG.   (0151-474 9626)

Further Reading

The following is a list of a few useful books. More reading material on specific topics can be obtained from the majority of the groups and organisations listed in Appendices 1 and 2.

Angelo, J. *Your Healing Power*. Piatkus, London, 1994.

Blate, M. *How to Heal Yourself Using Hand Acupressure*. Routledge & Kegan Paul, London, 1983.

Botton, J.; Bloom, W. (eds.) *The Seeker's Guide: a New Age Resource Book*. Aquarian/Thorsons, London, 1992.

Boyce, M. *Zoroastrians*. Routledge & Kegan Paul, London, 1979.

Brohn, P. *Gentle Giants*. Century Hutchinson, London, 1987.

Brown, C. *Optimum Healing*. Rider, London, 1998.

Chaitow, L.; Martin, S. *World without AIDS*. Thorsons Publishers, Wellingborough (UK), 1988.

Charlton-Stokes, J. *Jennie's Little Book of Herbs and Spice Remedies*. Universal Press, Cambridge, n.d.

Cooper, D. *Light up Your Life*. Ashgrove Press, 1991.

Cooper, D. *Power of Inner Peace*. Piatkus, London, 1994.

Cooper, J. C. *An Illustrated Encyclopaedia of Traditional Symbols*. Thames & Hudson, London, 1978.

Cousins, N. *Anatomy of an Illness*. Bantam Books Inc., New York.

Curtis, S.; Fraser, R.; Kohler, I. *Neal's Yard Natural Remedies*. Arkana/Penguin Books, London, 1988.

Davies, B. *Rainbow Journey*. Hodder & Stoughton, London, 1998.

De Angelis, B. *You Can Make Love All the Time*. Dell Books, New York, 1987.

Dickenson, D. *How to Fortify your Immune System*. Arlington Books, London, 1984.

Duin, N. *Health Help Directory*. Bedford Square Press, London, 1990.

Ellis, E. *Pathway to Sunrise*. Horus Books, 1998.

Endacott, M. (consultant ed.) *Encyclopaedia of Complementary Therapies*. Carlton Books, London, 1996.

Fry, J. (ed.) *The Beecham Manual for Family Practice*. 3rd edn. MTB Press, Lancaster (UK).

Fulder, S. (ed.) *Handbook of Complementary Medicine*. 2nd edn.

Furth, G. *The Secret World of Drawings*. Sigo Press, Boston, 1988.

Gawain, S. *Creative Visualisation*. Bantam Books Inc., New York, 1985.

Gillanders, A. *Reflexology*. Jenny Lee Publications, UK, 1988.

Glouberman, D. *Life Changes, Life Choices*. Thorsons, London, 1989.

Gosling, N. *Successful Herbal Medicine*. Thorsons Publishers, Wellingborough (UK), 1985.

Greer, R.; Woodward, R. A. *The Book of Vitamins and Healthfood Supplements*. Souvenir Press, London, 1995.

Gregory, S.; Leonardo, B. *Conquering AIDS Now*. Tree of Life Publications, California, 1986.

Guiley, R. *The Dream Book*. Pocket Books, USA, 1994.

Guiley, R. *The Miracle of Prayers*. Pocket Books, USA, 1995.

Hawkins, F. H. *Human Factors in Flight*. Gower Technical Press, Aldershot (UK), 1987.

Hay, L. L. *You Can Heal Your Life*. Hay House, California, 1984.

Heron, J. *Catharsis in Human Development*. British Postgraduate Medical Federation, 33 Willman Street, London WC1N 3EJ, 1977.

Heron, J. *Co-counselling*. Human Potential Research Project, University of Surrey, Guildford (UK), 1979.

Holford, P. *The Whole Health Manual*. Thorsons Publishers, Wellingborough (UK).

Insler, S. *The Gathas of Zarathustra*. Alta Iranica Publishers, 1974.

Jampolsky, G. G. *Love is Letting Go of Fear*. Bantam Books Inc., London and New York, 1985.

Japary, A. *The Gathas, Our Guide: The Divine Songs of Zarathustra*. Ushta Inc. Publishers, PO Box 1260, Cypress, CA90630, USA, 1989.

Judith, A.   *Wheels of Life: a User's Guide to the Chakra System.* Llewellyn Publications, 1990.

Jung, C. G.   *Memories, Dreams, Reflections.* Oxford University Press, Oxford, 1963.

Kenton, L.; Kenton, S.   *Raw Energy.* Century Hutchinson, London, 1984.

Kilmartin, A.   *Cystitis.* Thorsons, London, 1997.

King, E. (ed.)   *HIV and AIDS Treatment Directory.* NAM Publications, 1995.

Kübler-Ross, E.   *On Death and Dying.* Tavistock Publications, London, 1970.

Kunz, K.; Kunz, E.   *The Complete Guide to Foot Reflexology.* Thorsons Publishers, Wellingborough (UK), 1982.

Le Shan, L.   *How to Meditate.* Turnstone Press, USA, 1983.

Le Shan, L.   *You Can Fight for Your Life.* Thorsons Publishers, Wellingborough (UK), 1984.

Lewis, A.   *Selenium.* Thorsons Publishers, Wellingborough (UK), 1983.

Luthe, A.; Schultz, J. W.   *Autogenic Training and Therapy*, vols 1–6. Grune & Stratton, New York, 1969.

McWhirter, J.   *The Practical Guide to Candida.*   All Hallows House Foundation, 1995.

Meek, J.   *How to Boost Your Immune System: the Nutrition Connection.* ION Press, UK.

Mindell, E.   *The Food Medicine Bible.* Souvenir Press, London, 1994.

Mindell, E.   *The Vitamin Bible.* Arlington Books, London, 1979.

North, B.; Crittenden, P.   *Stop Herpes Now.* Thorsons Publishers, Wellingborough (UK), 1985.

Pelletier, K. R.   *Mind as a Healer: Mind as a Slayer.* Delta Books, USA, 1977.

Pietroni, P.   *Holistic Living.* J. M. Dent & Sons, London, 1988.

Pietroni, P. C. (ed.)   *Reader's Digest Family Guide to Alternative Medicine.* The Reader's Digest Association, London, 1991.

Proto, L.   *Self-Healing.* Piatkus Books, London, 1990.

Raphaell, K.   *Crystal Enlightenment.* Aurora Press, USA, 1985.

Reed Gach, M. *Acupressure: how to cure common ailments the natural way*. Piatkus, London, 1993.

Roman, S. *Spiritual Growth*. H. J. Kramer, USA, 1989.

Segal, B. S. *Love, Medicine and Miracles*. Rider, London, 1986.

Serinus, J. (ed.) *Psychoimmunity and the Healing Process*. Celestial Arts, California, 1986.

Sharma, C. H. *The International Manual of Homoeopathy and Natural Medicine*. Thorsons Publishers, Wellingborough (UK), 1985.

Simonton, O. C.; Simonton, S. M. *Getting Well Again*. Bantam Books Inc., New York, 1988.

Taraporewala, I. J. S. *The Religion of Zarathustra*. Taraporewala Publishers, Bombay, 1979. (Available from Ushta Inc. Publishers, PO Box 1260, Cypress, CA90630, USA.)

Trimmer, E. *The Magic of Magnesium*. Thorsons Publishers Wellingborough (UK), 1987.

Twyman, J. F. *Emissary of Light*. Hodder & Stoughton, 1997.

Ullman, M.; Zimmerman, N. *Working with Dreams*. Aquarian Press, Wellingborough (UK), 1987.

Weekes, C. *Self Help for Your Nerves*. Angus & Robertson, London, 1962.

Weiner, M. A. *Maximum Immunity*. Gateway Books, Bath, Avon, 1986.

Index